Testimonials for

ADVANCING EXCELLENCE IN HEALTHCARE QUALITY

Advancing Excellence in Healthcare Quality: 40 Strategies for Improving Patient Outcomes and Providing, Safe, High-Quality Healthcare provides readers with insight into 40 strategies healthcare leaders can use to effect change. Dr. McAslan describes how a patient-centered approach to care can improve health outcomes, increase patient safety, and reduce medical errors. She examines each strategy by describing the system change, providing a rational for implementing the change, and summarizing the "bottom-line" benefit.

Written from the clinician's perspective, the book describes how a physician-led team can decrease the fragmentation of the healthcare system, use technology to optimize the coordination of care in the hospital and in the ambulatory setting to prevent readmissions, reduce medication errors, and encourage patients to take personal responsibility for their health.

Healthcare leaders will find the book to be a source of ideas for change, and the healthcare providers in their organizations will be able to implement the changes that will affect their patients. It's a book that deserves a wide audience.

SUSAN L. TURNEY, MD, MS, FACMPE, FACP
President and CEO, MGMA Medical Group Management Association
Englewood, CO

Dr. McAslan's, *Advancing Excellence in Healthcare Quality: 40 Strategies for Improving Patient Outcomes and Providing, Safe, High-Quality Healthcare* is the essential checklist for improving quality of care, whether in the hospital or the ambulatory setting. She provides an easy-to-use structured approach to the most common quality issues faced by healthcare providers. It is an indispensable read for those starting a quality improvement program and for those who want to improve an existing quality program.

LAWRENCE SHAPIRO, MD
Formerly, Managed Care Director for the Palo Alto Medical Foundation
Author, *Quality Care, Affordable Care: How Physicians Can Reduce Variation and Lower Healthcare Costs*
Cupertino, CA

Advancing Excellence in Healthcare Quality: 40 Strategies for Improving Patient Outcomes and Providing, Safe, High-Quality Healthcare is more than just that. This book is packed with suggestions on how to improve the quality of healthcare. Many of the ideas are new, and integrating them into your everyday practice requires some thought. Read a section each day, follow the wise guidance from Dr. McAslan, and you will practice safer medicine.

KEVIN PHO, MD
Founder, KevinMD.com and Author, *Establishing, Managing and Protecting Your Online Reputation: A Social Media Guide for Physicians and Medical Practices*
Nashua, NH

Mary Sue McAslan has written a wonderfully practical book that is chock-full of helpful suggestions that healthcare professionals can put to work immediately. Focusing on patient-centered care, McAslan looks at optimizing outcomes, reducing readmissions, minimizing medical errors, and promoting prevention. This book is well-timed to help practitioners during a period of rapid change in healthcare. It dovetails beautifully with another cultural change for healthcare organizations: the growth of social media, which allows practitioners to extend their reach outside the confines of the office visit to improve healthcare and lower costs.

SUSAN M. GAY, MA
President, Infobrand
Author, *Establishing, Managing and Protecting Your Online Reputation: A Social Media Guide for Physicians and Medical Practices*
Wayne, PA

Dr. McAslan has expertly refined her extensive experience in quality and safety into an immensely readable compilation of practical strategies to make our healthcare system safer and, ultimately, better. By structuring her book around the goals envisioned in the Affordable Care Act, she reaches out to readers in medical practice and hospital settings alike who deal each day with the impacts of this game-changing legislation. Whether it is discussing lean management, team approaches, or electronic health records and patient portals, Mary Sue keeps her compassionate yet practical focus on what readers with clinical and administrative responsibilities can do now to improve the quality of care for their patients and communities. Read this book and you will come away with doable strategies to optimize outcomes, reduce hospital readmissions, minimize medication errors, and promote the prevention of disease.

ELIZABETH W. WOODCOCK, MBA, FACMPE, CPC
Woodcock & Associates
Atlanta, GA

Advancing Excellence in Healthcare Quality

40 STRATEGIES FOR IMPROVING PATIENT OUTCOMES AND PROVIDING SAFE, HIGH-QUALITY HEALTHCARE

Mary Sue McAslan, Pharm. D

Foreword by DAVID B. NASH, MD, MBA

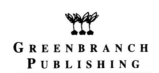

GREENBRANCH
PUBLISHING

13   8 7 6 5 4 3 2 1

Copyedited, typeset, indexed, and printed in the United States of America

PUBLISHER
Nancy Collins

EDITORIAL ASSISTANT
Jennifer Weiss

BOOK DESIGNER
Laura Carter
Carter Publishing Studio

INDEX
Robert Saigh

COPYEDITOR
Patricia George

TABLE OF CONTENTS

DEDICATION

To the four generations of healthcare professionals in my family who have provided high quality, patient-centered care in the past and will continue to do so for many years to come.

ACKNOWLEDGMENTS

I would like to acknowledge the many healthcare professionals with whom I have had the honor to work over the past 30 years and continue to work with on and day-to-day basis. It is through their hard work, dedication, and tireless efforts that our patients have received and will continue to receive high-quality and efficient healthcare.

I would also like to thank my "support staff," and especially my husband, Keith, who always seems to have just the right dose of advice at the right time; my children, Chip, Katie, John; and granddaughter, Liv, for all of their love and encouragement.

A special thanks goes to Nancy Collins, publisher, Greenbranch Publishing, for her passion and enthusiasm for healthcare quality and for providing me with the opportunity to make this book a reality.

ABOUT THE AUTHOR

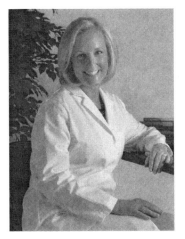

Mary Sue McAslan is a doctor of pharmacy specializing in medication safety and healthcare quality improvement. Dr. McAslan led her first quality circle in 1981 at North Mississippi Medical Center and has since gone on to lead quality improvement initiatives at the Cleveland Clinic Healthcare System, Kaiser Permanente, the Veteran's Healthcare Administration, and Omnicare, Inc.

In her current role as a lean six-sigma black belt, she provides leadership for root cause analysis teams, rapid process improvement teams, 5S initiatives and other Lean process improvement strategies.

Dr. McAslan has led efforts to improve patient outcomes, focusing on patient-centered medical homes, telemedicine clinics, and improved discharge planning. She has hands-on experience with one of the most comprehensive health information systems, including computerized physician order entry, e-prescribing, patient portals, clinical decision support tools, and medication reconciliation.

Dr. McAslan is the author of *Read the Prescription Label: and other tips to prevent deadly and costly medication errors* and the Personal Health System, available from Amazon or at www.drmarysue.com. Contact her directly at www.drmarysue.com.

Foreword

THIS IS NOT YOUR FATHER'S TEXTBOOK on quality and safety! Although several excellent textbooks on quality and safety are available, I wasn't sure the marketplace was ready for Mary Sue McAslan—boy, was I wrong!

McAslan, herself a pharmacist, has been toiling in the quality and safety field for three decades, largely unheralded, yet in her heartfelt style, she has delivered the goods.

Her book is divided into four main areas of focus, including optimizing outcomes, reducing readmissions, minimizing medication errors, and promoting disease prevention. Each of the four areas, then, has 10 specific, practical solutions that can be implemented almost immediately. This is the core strength of McAslan's work: a no-nonsense approach to a field that has more than its share of nonsense over the past 30 years.

Any practitioner, including doctors, nurses, pharmacists, and physicians' assistants, could take the information from this book and improve what they do the very next day. It is an easy read with almost a checklist quality to the recommendations. There is no barrier to entry in getting the work done because McAslan's style is so easy to understand: no complex formulas, no impossible-to-read flow diagrams, no arcane Pareto analyses, just solid advice about what to do with our next patients so that their care is of a higher quality and certainly is less prone to error.

Who should read this book? I believe McAslan has created just the right recipe that would appeal to the tastes of nearly everyone. That is, the book is appropriate for nurses, pharmacists, practice managers, hospital administrators, and physicians' assistants. In fact, it would be the perfect introductory text for an interprofessional attack on these issues. Given the current emphasis on team training and interprofessional training, McAslan has written the right book at the right time.

Finally, I was impressed with McAslan's "can-do" attitude. There didn't seem to be any problem too complex that could not be further elucidated into its component parts and therefore readily tackled tomorrow. She has an uncanny ability to simplify the work of many others who have gone before her in a way that is easy to digest.

Kudos to McAslan. I hope that *Advancing Excellence in Healthcare Quality* gets the wide readership that it so richly deserves. I only wish her book had come around earlier so we could recommend it to every trainee!

DAVID B. NASH, MD, MBA
Dean
The Raymond C. and Doris N. Grandon
Professor of Health Policy
Jefferson School of Population Health
Thomas Jefferson University
Philadelphia, PA

Introduction

DO YOU EVER FEEL THAT YOUR PATIENT'S CARE is spiraling out of your control?

Do you feel that your patient's care is becoming so fragmented and that something important might get missed, slip through the cracks, or get delayed in unnecessary paperwork or claims?

Do you question why deadly medication errors continue to happen despite using the most advanced technology?

Do you question why readmission rates are so high?

Do you wonder why patients continue to succumb to preventable chronic illnesses with decades of data supporting healthy lifestyles?

Do you wonder if there is anything that you can do about it?

THE IOM REPORT—FIFTEEN YEARS LATER

During the 30 years that I have been a clinical pharmacist specializing in the prevention of medication errors and the improvement of patient safety, I have seen many "quality improvement initiatives" in our healthcare organizations. Strategies aimed at reducing errors and improving safety were common in the 1980s and 1990s, but never seemed to impact the overall quality of care our patients were receiving. Unfortunately, many of these quality initiatives did not result in positive measurable, sustained change.

In 1999, the Institute of Medicine (IOM) published the oft-cited report "To Err is Human: Building a Safer Health System," which stated

> Health care in the United States is not as safe as it should be--and can be. At least 44,000 people, and perhaps as many as 98,000 people die in hospitals each year as a result of medical errors that could have been prevented, according to estimates from two major studies. Even using the lower estimate, preventable medical errors in hospitals exceed attributable deaths to such feared threats as motor-vehicle wrecks, breast cancer, and AIDS. (1)

Have we made measurable change since 1999? Are medical errors decreasing? Are readmission rates lower? Are costs of care lower? Are we more efficient?

My perspective, from working with frustrated, confused patients on a day-to-day basis and reviewing numerous chronic, preventable medical errors, is that we are not doing a better job. It is my opinion that we, as a country, have seen very little progress toward changing the results of the IOM report. Why is it that we are no closer today to solving this healthcare dilemma than we were in 1999?

WHY THE IOM REPORT DIDN'T GET RESULTS

The IOM report gave healthcare providers and hospital administrators, for the first time, a very clear and public picture of the dismal state of healthcare quality in America. Patients were dying every day in our hospitals as a result of preventable medical errors, which were due in large part to the poor quality of care. The IOM report also gave providers and administrators every statistic, fact, and figure needed to prove that we were in deep trouble regarding patient safety and quality. Every chart and graph in this report clearly depicted every mistake and unnecessary dollar spent in paying for these mistakes. The IOM report left no question that we needed to do something fast to change the course of healthcare in this country. But once the initial outrage faded and the government moved on to other "more burning" issues, the IOM report faded from the limelight.

What was left undone by the IOM report was *how* we were supposed to address these findings on a grass roots level. Of course, there were government programs initiated to improve outcomes and reduce costs, but the average healthcare provider was still faced with the fragmentation, duplication, and frustration of everyday medical practice.

THE TIME IS NOW

On March 23, 2010, President Obama signed the Patient Protection and Affordable Care Act (also called the Affordable Care Act, AFA, Obamacare) into law. This law is meant to put into place comprehensive reforms aimed at improving access to affordable healthcare and protection from abusive insurance company practices.

What the passing of the Affordable Care Act actually translates into remains to be seen, but what is apparent is that we now have national impetus to improve the quality of healthcare in America. There are many questions surrounding the overall plan, including the integrity of the infrastructure to support this change, how coordinated and interoperable these changes will be, and the rationality of the pace of implementation. But what the Affordable Care Act does represent is a step in the right direction for healthcare quality, and this book supports those efforts with initiatives to use in your practices and institutions.

WHY THIS BOOK

This book presents 40 basic, practical strategies that I use in my day-to-day hospital practice to help improve the quality of care for my patients. I wrote the book not as a panacea, but as an overview of the different systems and solutions that are available to practices and hospitals today. Not all strategies are appropriate for all providers, practices, or hospitals, but some will apply to you. Start with one initiative, stick with it until it is successfully implemented, reach your goals, and then move on to the next initiative. Keep going until your practice or hospital has achieved the level of performance that you are satisfied with and proud of.

You are not alone in this journey. The changes that have been legislated by the Affordable Care Act have come hard and fast. They represent a sea change, especially for those providers who do not have the resources of large healthcare systems and/or who practice in remote, rural settings. This book represents my experience with some successful systems and solutions and, I hope, my experience with them will be of benefit to you.

THE FOUR AREAS OF FOCUS

Four areas of the Affordable Care Act have been designated as being instrumental in improving the quality of care.

These are:
1. Optimizing Outcomes
2. Reducing Readmissions
3. Minimizing Medication Errors
4. Promoting Disease Prevention.

This book is divided into these four sections and offers 10 different practical solutions in each section to implement in your practice or hospital setting.

1. Optimize Outcomes

Optimize Outcomes reviews the Stage 1 and Stage 2 Meaningful Use measures, including electronic health records, e-prescribing, clinical decision support, summaries of care, and clinical quality measures. This section provides actionable strategies for providers in private practice as well as health system administrators that will help meet the requirements of Stage 2 Meaningful Use.

2. Reduce Readmissions

Reduce Readmission approaches care from the patient-centered model. The section addresses working collaboratively with patients and caregivers from the hospital admission, through the discharge process, and into the ambulatory setting. New strategies such as patient-centered medical home care, telemedicine, chronic disease management, and tactics for ensuring medication adherence are presented.

3. Minimize Medication Errors

Minimize Medication Errors presents the concept of the blame-free institution or a just culture. This describes the hospital or healthcare setting that recognizes that even the most competent professionals will make mistakes but that they should not be held accountable for system failures. A just culture also has zero tolerance for reckless behavior. This section includes topics related to adverse drug events, drug interactions, high-risk medications, and patient name mix-ups. It concludes with a discussion of problem analysis techniques including root cause analysis and lean process improvement.

4. Promote Prevention

Promote Prevention provides clinicians with strategies to inspire wellness in their patients. The section addresses weight management, lowering blood pressure, smoking cessation, and diabetes prevention. This section also addressed the issues surrounding health literacy and the social determinants of health.

COMMON THEME—THE TEAM APPROACH

The physician has and will maintain ultimate decision-making responsibility for his or her patients' care. The physician is the captain of the ship. However, the captain can't sail the ship by him or herself. No ship can leave port without a complete and coordinated crew. Each of the sections of this book circles back to one common theme: team-based care.

Enabling well-trained healthcare professionals, including physician assistants, nurse practitioners, pharmacists, and nurses, to take some of the responsibility for patient care off the shoulders of the physician will promote improved communication and coordination of care for our patients. Once this is done, providers can rely on the excellence in their healthcare staff and start taking back the control of their patients' care. Providers can begin to decrease the fragmentation and streamline care by maximizing the technology available to them, optimize the coordination of care in the hospital and in the ambulatory setting to prevent readmissions, improve systems to reduce deadly and costly medication errors, and work with patients to inspire wellness and prevent chronic disease.

This represents a new and improved team approach that replaces the old, siloed approach to medical care. The team approach to patient care is the key to reducing fragmentation and improving care coordination. If you are truly serious about improving the quality of your patient's care, then let's get to work.

Reference

1. Institute of Medicine. *To Err Is Human: Building a Safer Health System.* Washington, DC: National Academy Press. 2000.

Optimize Outcomes

*Quality is never an accident; it is always
the result of high intention, sincere effort, intelligent
direction and skillful execution; it represents
the wise choice of many alternatives.*

—WILLIAM A. FOSTER

CHAPTER 1

The EHR Evolution

According to the Centers for Medicare and Medicaid Services (CMS), certified electronic health record technology used in a meaningful way is one piece of a broader health information technology infrastructure needed to reform the healthcare system in the United States and improve healthcare quality and efficiency, and patient safety.

The electronic health record (EHR) is a longitudinal electronic record of patient health information. This information is compiled by one or more encounters in any healthcare delivery setting. The information in the EHR includes patient demographics, progress notes, problems, medications, vital signs, past medical history, immunizations, laboratory data, and radiology reports. (1)

Electronic health records require an investment of time and resources; however the Medicare and Medicaid EHR Incentive Programs through the Health Information Technology for Economic and Clinical Health Act (HITECH), provide incentive payments to eligible professionals, eligible hospitals, and critical access hospitals as they adopt, implement, upgrade, or demonstrate meaningful use of certified EHR technology. Eligible professionals can receive up to $44,000 through the Medicare EHR Incentive Program, and up to $63,750 through the Medicaid EHR Incentive Program. (2)

MEANINGFUL USE OF ELECTRONIC HEALTH RECORDS

The goal of HITECH is to achieve significant improvements in patient care (i.e., meaningful use) by using electronic health records. In 2010, the Centers for Medicare and Medicaid Services (CMS) published the final rule regarding the EHR incentive program. This rule specified the criteria eligible providers (EPs), eligible hospitals, and critical access hospitals (CAHs) must meet to qualify for an incentive payment. In that rule, CMS described three different stages of meaningful use requirements for EHRs, with each stage requiring the increasing use of EHRs and information exchange. Meaningful use will evolve in these three stages:

Stage 1: 2011–2012: Data capture and sharing

Stage 2: 2016: Advance clinical processes

Stage 3: Will initiate 2017 and focus on improved outcomes

Stage 1 and Stage 2 EHR Objectives and Measures

OBJECTIVE: Record the following demographics: preferred language, gender, race, ethnicity, and date of birth.

> **Stage 1 Measure:** More than 50% of all unique patients seen by the EP have demographics recorded as structured data.

> **Stage 2 Measure:** More than 80% of all unique patients seen by the EP have demographics recorded as structured data.

OBJECTIVE: Record and chart changes in height, weight, blood pressure (ages 3 and over); calculate and display BMI; plot and display growth charts for patients ages 1–20 years, including BMI.

> **Stage 1 Measure:** More than 50% of all unique patients ages 2 and over seen by the EP have blood pressure, height, and weight recorded as structured data.

> **Stage 2 Measure:** More than 80% of all unique patients seen by the EP have blood pressure (for patients ages 3 and over only), and height and weight (all ages) recorded as structured data.

OBJECTIVE: Incorporate clinical lab test results into certified EHR technology as structured data.

> **Stage 1 Measure:** More than 40% of all clinical lab test results ordered by the EP during the EHR reporting period that are in a positive/negative or numerical format are incorporated in certified EHR technology as structured data.

> **Stage 2 Measure:** More than 55% of all clinical lab test results ordered by the EP during the EHR reporting period that are in a positive/negative or numerical format are incorporated in certified EHR technology as structured data.

OBJECTIVE: Generate lists of patients by specific conditions to use for quality improvement, reduction of disparities, research, or outreach.

> **Stage 1 Measure:** Generate at least one report listing patients of the EP who have a specific condition.

> **Stage 2 Measure:** Generate at least one report listing patients of the EP who have a specific condition.

OBJECTIVE: Use clinically relevant information to identify patients who should receive reminders for preventive/follow-up care.

Stage 1 Measure: More that 20% of all unique patients 65 years of age or older or 5 years of age or younger are sent an appropriate reminder during the EHR reporting period.

Stage 2 Measure: EHR is used to identify and provide reminders for preventive/follow-up care for more than 10% of patients who had two or more office visits in the past two years.

OBJECTIVE: Be able to submit electronic data to immunization registries or immunization information systems and actual submission except where prohibited and in accordance with applicable law and practice.

Stage 1 Measure: Perform at least one test of certified EHR technology's capacity to submit electronic data to immunization registries and follow-up submission if the test is successful (unless none of the immunization registries to which the EP submits such information have the capacity to receive the information electronically).

Stage 2 Measure: Successful ongoing submission of electronic immunization data from certified EHR technology to an immunization registry or immunization information system for the entire EHR reporting period.

OBJECTIVE: Protect electronic health information created or maintained by the certified EHR technology through the implementation of appropriate technical capabilities.

Stage 1 Measure: Conduct or review a security risk analysis and implement security updates as necessary and correct identified security deficiencies as part of the risk management process.

Stage 2 Measure: Conduct or review a security risk analysis that includes addressing the encryption/security of data at rest, and implement security updates as necessary and correct identified security deficiencies as part of the risk management process.

THE CONS OF ELECTRONIC HEALTH RECORDS

The meaningful use objectives related to electronic health records may be the catalyst needed to begin the process toward widespread use of health information technology; however, these admirable goals may be a bit overzealous. Each of the seven goals above requires a great deal of resources and time, and tying the implementation of these goals to unrealistic timelines may be setting providers up to fail.

A recent survey shows that in 2010, only 2% of U. S. hospitals reported having EHRs that would allow them to meet meaningful use criteria. (3) My personal experience with one of the oldest and most comprehensive electronic health record systems in the United States prompts me to caution against implementing too large a system too quickly. Although electronic records may be available to all providers in an institution, certain demographic data, clinical decision support, and clinical reminders may be underused or omitted entirely.

Additionally, patient portals that offer educational and communication opportunities may be a daunting obstacle for patients who have limited computer literacy or who do not own a computer. Providers who are in the process of implementing EHRs may want to start with a simple system that can be added to and modified as staff becomes more fluent and comfortable with the complexities of the system.

THE PROS OF ELECTRONIC HEALTH RECORDS

The benefits of EHRs include providing information about patient history, prior allergic or adverse reactions, and drug interactions. EHRs help verify medications and dosages and reduce the risk of unnecessary tests and procedures. Providers who use EHRs are better able to coordinate the care they deliver with other providers. EHRs also can help patients and their caregivers take part more fully in their healthcare decisions by using the patient portals. (4)

The benefits of EHRs also include improved medical practice management through improved practice efficiencies and cost savings. (5) According to a national survey of doctors: (6)

- 79% of providers report that with an EHR, their practices function more efficiently.
- 82% report that sending prescriptions electronically (e-prescribing) saves time.
- 68% of providers see their EHR as an asset with recruiting physicians.
- 75% say they receive lab results faster.
- 70% report enhanced data confidentiality.

EHRs have been shown to improve medical practice management and create more efficient practices by integrating scheduling systems that link appointments directly to progress notes, automate coding, and manage claims. They provide time savings by centralizing chart management and enhancing communication with staff, other providers, and labs. Many EHRs provide automated drug formulary checks by health plans, decreasing time spent with pharmacies determining the appropriate formulary equivalent agent. (3)

EHRs affect revenue generation by reducing the time and resources necessary for manual charge entry, resulting in more accurate billing and a reduction in lost charges. EHRs also reduce charge lag days and vendor/insurance denials associated with late filing and minimize claims requiring Advance Beneficiary Notice. (3) EHRs reduce administrative tasks, such as filling out forms and processing billing requests, which leads to more streamlined processed and reduced costs.

EHRS—ARE WE THERE YET?

- The EHR evolution is a long arduous task. Plan to create an "adaptive reserve" of time, energy, and resources. Devote time to reviewing what went right and what went wrong for ongoing training programs and troubleshooting. Do not think that you can do this while patients are waiting to be seen.
- Train "super-users." These are members of your staff who are interested in becoming experts in the new computer system. They will help troubleshoot any problems and help train new staff members. They will also be the valuable link to the computer system manufacturer.
- Using the computer system for panel management as defined by the meaningful use criteria may be difficult. Be sure to get this clarified with your EHR systems developer before assuming that your system has these capabilities.
- If you believe you need to hire an IT specialist to conduct the security risk analysis, do so; however, you may wish to use a template to help identify security weaknesses. A template is available from the Office of the National Coordinator's Risk Analysis Tool (www.healthit.gov).

BOTTOM LINE

Meaningful use is defined as using EHR technology to improve quality, safety, and efficiency to reduce health disparities. EHRs can be used to improve care coordination and engage patients and their families in their healthcare as well as provide privacy and security of health information. However, it may take many years to successfully implement an electronic health record system in your facility or office.

References

1. EHR. HIMSS. http://www.HIMSS.org. Accessed January 21, 2013.
2. Centers for Medicare and Medicaid Services. EHR incentive programs. Centers for Medicare and Medicaid Services. *http://www.cms.gov*. Accessed January 21, 2013.
3. Jha A, DesRoches CM, Kralovec MD, Joshi, MS. A progress report on electronic health records in US hospitals. *Health AFF*. October 2010: 29(10): 1951–1957. Doi: 10.1377/hlthaff.2010.0502

4. HealthIT.gov. Why adopt EHRs? HealthIT.gov. *http://www.healthit.gov/providers-professionals/why-adopt-ehrs*. Accessed January 21, 2013.

5. HealthIT.gov Benefits of EHRs—Medical practice efficiencies and cost savings. HealthIT.gov. *http://healthit.gov/providers-professionals/medical-practice-efficiencies-cost-savings*. Accessed January 21, 2013.

6. 4. Jamoom E, Patel V, et al. *National perceptions of EHR adoption: Barriers, benefits, and federal policies.* Presented at the National Conference on Health Statistics, August 2012.

7. 9. HealthIT.gov. Security risk assessment tool. HealthIT.gov. *http://www.healthit.gov/security-risk-assessment-tool*. Accessed January 21, 2013.

CHAPTER 2

The CPOE Solution

COMPUTERIZED PHYSICIAN ORDER ENTRY (CPOE) helps eliminate hand-written orders and reduces errors related to medication prescribing by improving legibility and completeness. (1) CPOE offers clinical decision support and references to evidence-based protocols and guidelines. These systems speed order transmission to pharmacy, lab, radiology, and other services.

Studies of CPOE systems have shown a positive impact on transcription-related medication errors. An epidemiology study of prescribing errors found a rate of 62.4 errors per 1000 medication orders. (2) Of these errors, 31% were considered clinically significant and 64% were determined preventable with CPOE. In addition, 43% of prescribing errors that were previously classified as potentially harmful to the patient were determined likely to be preventable with CPOE (2)

The Centers for Medicare and Medicaid Services (CMS) includes the use of CPOE in Stage 2 Meaningful Use for eligible professionals (EPs).

Stage 1 Objective: Use CPOE for medication orders directly entered by any licensed healthcare professional who can enter orders into the medical record per state, local, and professional guidelines.

Stage 1 Measure: More than 30% of unique patients with at least one medication in their medication list seen by the EP have at least one medication order entered using CPOE.

Stage 2 Objective: Use CPOE for medication, laboratory, and radiology orders directly entered by licensed healthcare professionals who can enter orders into the medical record per state, local, and professional guidelines to create the first record of the order.

Stage 2 Measure: More than 60% of medication, 30% of laboratory, and 30% of radiology orders created by the EP during the electronic health record (EHR) reporting period are recorded using CPOE.

ADVANTAGES OF CPOE

Using CPOE to order medications provides an automatic double-check against relevant patient information. Drug–drug interactions, therapeutic duplication, drug allergies, lab values, and dose checks are just some of the ways CPOE helps prevent medication errors. CPOE also provides a safer way to order medications because it alleviates handwritten prescriptions. Legibility issues, which have caused medication errors for many years, are no longer an issue. CPOE also reduces the chance of selecting a drug that is not on the health plan's formulary, or one that is not appropriate for the patient.

Additional advantages include: prescriptions reach the pharmacy faster; prescriptions may be less subject to error due to look-alike drug names; the use of apothecary measures and unacceptable abbreviations may decrease; identification of the prescribing physician is easier; there's an ability to link to adverse drug event reporting system; ability to avoid trailing zeros (5.0) and utilization of leading zeros (0.5); there's an ability to link to order sets and protocols and to formulary recommendations. Lastly, CPOE provides an up-to-date list of the patient's medical record, including all medications, that is readily accessible for all practitioners to view at follow-up visits.

DISADVANTAGES OF CPOE

Despite the numerous advantages of CPOE, there remain concerns that it may actually cause some medication errors. In a recent study published in *JAMA* (3), 22 different situations were identified in which CPOE increased the risk of prescribing errors. These errors fell under two categories: 1) Information errors (fragmentation and systems integration failures) and 2) human–machine interface flaws (machine rules that do not correspond to work organization or usual behaviors). These errors included:

Information Errors:
- Assumption that displayed doses were dosing guidelines when in fact these were based on pharmacy's purchasing requirements.
- Failure to discontinue medications, leading to "double doses," duplicate therapy, and interactions.
- Failure to discontinue medications ordered with procedures and tests when the procedure/test was canceled.
- Failure to discontinue NOW and as-needed orders.
- Failure to renew antibiotics.
- Expectation that physicians know which diluents to order with IVs.
- Overriding allergy information.
- Overriding conflicting or duplicative medications.

Human-Machine Interface Errors:
- Improper log on or log off

- Selecting the wrong patient.
- Selecting the wrong medication from the drug menu.
- Failure to restart medications post-operatively.
- Orders that are entered late in the day are "lost" for 24 hours.
- Cumbersome charting of administered meds for nursing staff.
- Inflexibility of system when attempting to order non-formulary medications.

With more hospitals implementing CPOE systems, providers must be aware of the pitfalls in this technology and the errors that it may cause.

SUCCESSFUL CPOE STRATEGIES

- Implementing a CPOE system effectively requires that medical staff learn about, train on, and use the new system. Include physician champions (super-users) to instruct peers during the implementation process. Involve the physician super-users and chief residents in the training of new residents and continually update residents about any new additions or changes to the system.
- Include regular evaluation and feedback by all users to reduce barriers to appropriate utilization. Chronic work-arounds or refusals to use the system should be red flags that the technology (or training) is not meeting the needs of the staff.
- Include strategies for dealing with unexpected situations (e.g., power outages) and down time.
- Ensure that the EHR system has codified medications. Without using codified medications you will be at risk of failing the meaningful use criteria. Look for an EHR with a pre-loaded medication database, which makes choosing a codified medication for updating medication lists and e-prescribing an easy and efficient process.
- Many of the safety benefits attributed to CPOE may be completely lost when providers override system alerts. Clinical decision support systems such as medication allergy alerts, duplicate drug therapy, wrong doses, and drug interactions are errors that are preventable with proper use of CPOE.

BOTTOM LINE

- As more hospitals implement CPOE systems to meet the Stage 2 Meaningful Use measures, providers must be aware of the associated risks and proactively address ways to prevent errors while maximizing the benefits of this new technology.

References

1. Forni, A. Chu H, Fanikos J. Technology utilization to prevent medication errors. *Curr Drug Saf.* January 2010: 5(1):13–8.

2. Bobb A, Gleason K, Husch M, et al. The epidemiology of prescribing errors: The potential impact of computerized prescriber order entry. *Arch Intern Med.* 164(7):782-792. Doi: 10.1001archinte164.7.785.

3. Koppel R, Metlay J, et al. Role of computerized physician order entry systems in facilitating medication errors. *JAMA.* 293(10):1197–1203.

CHAPTER 3

Can I Have Some Support Please?

CLINICAL DECISION SUPPORT SYSTEMS (CDSS) provide clinicians with patient-specific information at the point of care. CDSS helps providers select appropriate medication therapy, preventing drug interactions, duplication of therapy, allergic reactions, or other adverse events. More sophisticated CDSS combine real-time patient data, such as age, weight, and renal and hepatic function, with evidence-based therapeutic recommendations to prevent dosing errors and improve patient safety. Clinical decision support also includes automatic routine reminders for preventative measures such as immunizations, smoking cessation, and weight management.

Automated clinical alerts represent an important part of current error reduction strategies that help to reduce the cost and improve the quality and safety of healthcare delivery. (1) CDSS links to formularies, guidelines, order sets, and dosing calculators for assistance with appropriate medication selection.

The Centers for Medicare and Medicaid Services (CMS) has included Clinical Decision Support in Stage 1 and 2 Meaningful Use measures for eligible professionals (EPs).

Stage 1 Objective: Implement one clinical decision support rule relevant to specialty or high clinical priority along with the ability to track compliance with that rule.

Stage 1 Measure: Implement one clinical decision support rule.

Stage 2 Objective: Use clinical decision support to improve performance on high-priority health conditions.

Stage 2 Measures:
1. Five clinical decision support interventions related to four or more clinical quality measures, if applicable, have been implemented at a relevant point in patient care for the entire electronic health record (EHR) reporting period; and
2. The EP, eligible hospital or CAH has enabled the functionality for drug–drug and drug–allergy interaction checks for the entire EHR reporting period.

It is important to remember that the ultimate safety and effectiveness of technology depends on the capability of human users; any form of technology can have adverse effects if not operated within a safe workflow process. (4) In 2008, the United States Joint Commission on Accreditation of Healthcare Organizations issued a *Sentinel Event Alert* entitled "Safely implementing health information and converging technologies." This alert brings to light the safety risks and preventable adverse events that technology implementation can create or perpetuate.

According to the Joint Commission, unintended adverse events typically stem from human–machine interfaces or organization/system design. (3) Physicians have reported a loss of professional autonomy when clinical decision support systems prevent ordering medications they require or force the use of clinical guidelines that may not apply to their patient. Clinicians also report "alert fatigue" from systems that generate excessive numbers of potentially irrelevant drug safety alerts. This "alert fatigue" leads to clinicians ignoring even the most important alerts and, to override them, potentially impacting patient safety. (4)

CDSS helps provide information related to best practices, clinical standards, and guidelines, as well as alerts to assist with prevention and other health issues. However, while the CDSS tools are helpful, they are only as good as the data programmed into them. Clinicians should ensure that the data are updated regularly and reflect current practices. Lastly, clinicians should be aware that these tools are merely a form of transmitting information on best practices and should always be used to supplement, not replace, the clinicians' own best judgment. (2)

THE CDSS SOLUTION

- Create a CDSS that is automatic, provides suggestions at a time and location where the decisions are being made, and provides actionable recommendations. (5)
- Create a CDSS of tiered safety alerts that informs providers of the urgency and relevancy of the alert. Decide which alerts will require a "hard stop" and require documentation before proceeding.
- Ensure that patient information is current and accurate (i.e., medication lists, allergies, and adverse reactions). Wrong patient information will trigger frequent and inaccurate CDSS alerts.
- Ensure that the information embedded in the CDSS is current and accurate. This includes new drugs, treatments, and updated clinical guidelines.
- Eliminate all dangerous abbreviations and dose designations from CDSS tools, including U, IU, QD, QOD, QID, MS, MSO4, and MgS04.
- Ensure that CDSS are integrated into the physician's cognitive workflow and that the safety aspects of these systems do not increase time to care for patients. This may decrease, not increase, the physician's motivation to use these systems. (5)

- If a provider is going to override the recommendation/notification of the CDSS, require mandatory documentation to justify the override of the alert.
- Ensure that alerts are created and addressed when necessary without inducing "alert fatigue." Overriding alerts and reminders is a common problem and systems need to be designed with alert criticality in mind.
- Prior to implementation of any healthcare technology, create a training program for all staff members who will use it, including clinicians, pharmacists, nurses, medical residents, locum tenens, etc., and provide frequent updates to ensure staff stays current with new software or changes.
- Prior to implementation, ensure that all standardized order sets and guidelines are tested on paper and approved by the Pharmacy and Therapeutics (P&T) Committee. Require that the P&T Committee review and approve all electronic order sets and clinical decision support alerts on a routine basis.

BOTTOM LINE

Clinical decision support systems, along with other forms of health information technology, can lead to reduced medication errors and improved patient care; however, these tools are meant to supplement, not replace critical thinking and clinical judgment.

References

1. Kuperman G. Medication-related clinical decision support in computerized provider order entry. *J Am Med Inform Assoc.* 2007. 13(4): 369–371.
2. American Medical Association. Clinical decision support tools. American Medical Association. http://www.ama-assn.org/ama/pub/physician-resources/practice-management-center/health-insurer-payer-relations/clinical-integrity/clinical-decision-support-tools.page. Accessed November 24, 2012.
3. Weiner, JP. "e-iatrogenesis": The most critical unintended consequence of CPOE and other HIT. *J Am Med Inform Assoc.* 2007 May-June;14(3):387–388.
4. The Joint Commission. Sentinel event issue alert #42—safely implementing health information and converging technologies. The Joint Commission. http://jointcommission.org/assets/1/18/SEA_42.pdf. Accessed November 24, 2012.
5. Berner, ES. June 2009. Clinical decision support systems: State of the art. Agency for Healthcare Research and Quality No. 09-0069-EF. May 2012. http://healthit.ahrq.gov.

CHAPTER 4

The Future Is Now— e-Prescribing

ELECTRONIC PRESCRIBING OR E-PRESCRIBING (e-Rx) is the computer-based electronic transmission of a prescription. It takes the place of a hard-copy paper or faxed prescription and enhances the provider's ability to send accurate, error-free, and legible prescriptions directly to the pharmacy from the point of care. (1)

E-prescribing can greatly enhance patient safety. (2) It has been instrumental in reducing actual and potential medication errors, adverse drug reactions, and other adverse events. It can reduce costs by increasing compliance with formulary medications and increasing the use of generics or lower-cost alternative agents. E-prescribing can enable payers to communicate information to prescribers that may lead to improved quality and better patient experience, formulary alerts, safety alerts, adherence reminders, and gaps in care.

In addition to enhancing patient safety, e-prescribing can help save time and resources in the medical practice as well as the pharmacy. It can reduce the time spent making phone calls or faxing to pharmacies for prescription renewals, formulary substitutions, generic substitutions, and clarifications due to legibility issues. (2) A study by MGMA's Group Practice Network estimated that the time spent managing unnecessary administrative complications related to prescription costs nearly $15,700 annually for each full-time physician. (3)

Lastly, e-prescribing has been shown to improve medication compliance. In a study by IMS and Walgreens, e-prescribing resulted in an 11% increase in prescriptions reaching the pharmacy to be filled. (4)

E-PRESCRIBING AND MEANINGFUL USE

E-prescribing is one of the more successful aspects of meaningful use. It is one of the key action items in the government's plan to facilitate the implementation of electronic medical records and a national electronic health information plan in the United States. (1) Several Stage 1 and 2 Meaningful Use requirements are supported by e-prescribing. These include:

Objective: Generate and transmit permissible prescriptions electronically (e-Rx).

Stage 1 Measure: More than 40% of all permissible prescriptions written by the eligible provider (EP) are transmitted electronically using certified EHR technology (comparison to drug formulary is not included).

Stage 2 Measure: More than 50% of all permissible prescriptions, or all prescriptions written by the EP, are queried for a drug formulary and transmitted electronically using certified EHR technology.

Exclusion Criteria

CMS recognizes that some providers practice in areas where electronic prescribing may be limited. CMS allows those providers to claim exclusion to this measure if they do not have a pharmacy within their organization or within 10 miles of the provider's practice location that can accept electronic prescriptions.

E-PRESCRIBING OF CONTROLLED SUBSTANCES

In June 2010, the Drug Enforcement Agency (DEA) issued an interim final rule allowing e-prescribing of controlled substances. This represented a breakthrough that gave prescribers the additional option of transmitting prescriptions for Schedule II–Schedule V controlled substances electronically rather than written, manually signed, or oral prescriptions. (2)

To electronically transmit prescriptions for controlled substances to pharmacies, providers must take certain steps. These include:

- The prescriber must use an e-prescribing application certified for electronic prescribing of controlled substances (EPCS).
- The prescriber must complete an ID-proofing process conducted by credential service providers or certification authorities approved by the federal government.
- The prescriber must use a "two-factor authentication" credential each and every time he or she issues a prescription for a controlled substance. Authentication credentials include the following:
  - ✓ Something you *know*: password, PIN
  - ✓ Something you *have*: hard token separate from computer being accessed
  - ✓ Something you *are*: any biometric that meets the DEA's requirements

COSTS RELATED TO E-PRESCRIBING

Costs of e-prescribing can vary depending on the type of system selected. Electronic health record systems that include e-prescribing can be more comprehensive but can also be more costly than stand-alone systems. However, initial cost is only one part of the equation. (2) Vendor fees, training, temporary decrease in productivity due to training or workflow redesign, practice management interfaces, customization, maintenance upgrades, and data conversion may all represent unforeseen "costs" to e-prescribing implementation. Ultimately, all costs should be compared to the expected benefits such as improved efficiency and productivity of the physician practice. (2)

E-RX

- E-prescribing represents a more efficient, accurate, and safer method of prescribing medications by replacing hard-copy, manually written paper prescriptions with secure information exchange between providers and pharmacies.
- When you are e-prescribing, it is essential that you have a codified medication list in the EHR system. Without this, you will be at risk for failing the e-prescribing measure. Be sure the EHR comes with a pre-loaded medication database, making e-prescribing quick and accurate.
- E-prescribing is a key factor in implementing and meeting Stage 1 and Stage 2 Meaningful Use requirements.
- The DEA permits prescription for controlled substances to be issued as long as regulatory requirements are met.

BOTTOM LINE

E-prescribing is a convenient, accurate, safe method of generating, transmitting, and filling a prescription. It reduces risks for the provider and patient by ensuring that complete and legible prescription information is sent directly from the healthcare provider to the pharmacy.

References

1. Centers for Medicare and Medicaid Services. E-prescribing. Centers for Medicare and Medicaid Services. *http://www.cms.gov/Medicare/E-Health/Eprescribing/index.html*. Accessed January 26, 2013.
2. American Medical Association. A clinician's guide to e-prescribing. American Medical Association. *http://www.ama-assn.org*. Accessed on January 26, 2013.
3. Medical Group Management Association. Analyzing the cost of administrative complexity in group practice. Medical Group Management Association. *http://www.mgma.com/about/about-mgma/about-center-for-research/analyzing-the-cost-of-administrative-complexity*. Published September 2004.
4. Walgreens and IMS. New research suggests that, when sent electronically, more new prescriptions make it from doctor's office to pharmacy to patient [press release]. Walgreens and IMS. October 15, 2007.

CHAPTER 5

Staying Connected— Patient Portals

PATIENT PORTALS ARE ONLINE HEALTHCARE applications that look like a website at first glance, but really are much more. (1) Portals allow patients to obtain information and to interact and communicate with their healthcare providers. These portals enable patients to log in and view their medical history and lab results. They provide a means to request prescription renewals and specialty referrals. They assist with appointment scheduling and online bill payment, and provide a secure method for a two-way patient–provider communications.

Patient portals add efficiencies that providers and their staffs need to better manage their practices and improve patient access and care. Portals offer the convenience of 24/7 self-service for patients and the option for staff to respond at a time most convenient for them. Patient portals are also helpful for practices trying to meet the federal government's criteria for meaningful use.

VIEW, DOWNLOAD, OR TRANSMIT

Objective: Provide patients with the ability to view online, download, and transmit their health information within four business days of the information being available to the EP.

Stage 1 Measure: More than 50% of all unique patients seen by the EP who request an electronic copy of their health information are provided it within three business days. This includes diagnostic test results, problem list, and medication allergies.

Stage 2a Measure: More than 50% of all unique patients seen by the EP during the EHR reporting period are provided timely (within four business days after the information is available to the EP) online access to their health information subject to the EP's discretion to withhold certain information.

Stage 2b Measure: More than 5% of all unique patients seen by the EP during the EHR reporting period (or their authorized representatives) view, download, or transmit their health information to a third party.

OBJECTIVE: Provide clinical summaries for patients for each office visit.

> **Stage 1 Measure:** Clinical summaries provided to patients for more than 50% of all office visits within three business days.

> **Stage 2 Measure:** Clinical summaries provided to patients within one business day for more than 50% of office visits.

OBJECTIVE: Use secure electronic messaging to communicate with patients about relevant health information.

> **Stage 2 Measure:** A secure message was sent using the electronic messaging function of the certified EHR technology by more than 5% of unique patients seen during the EHR reporting period.

Despite the fact that the implementation of patient portals has been limited to date, the requirements of Stage 2 Meaningful Use—that EPs ensure at least 5% of patients view, download, or transmit their electronic health records—may lead to a significant rise in their use. Although providers have expressed concern over meeting these standards, patients have shown that they will use portals if they include the features that they consider to be most valuable. (2)

Large organizations that use patient portals on a routine basis show that patients initially used patient portals to refill prescriptions, access facility directories, obtain educational materials and schedule appointments. As new features were added, patients were able to access lab results, refill prescriptions, and have electronic consultations with physicians. (3)

MYHEALTHEVET

The U.S. Department of Veterans Affairs (VA) Veterans Health Administration offers a patient portal called MyHealtheVet. (4) This portal system has three levels of account types: basic, advanced, and premium. The basic account provides limited access to features in My HealtheVet that the patient self-enters.

These include (self-reported):
- Activity journal
- Allergies
- Family health history
- Food journal
- Healthcare providers
- Health insurance
- Immunizations
- Labs and tests

- Medical events
- Medications and supplements
- Health history
- Current goals
- Completed goals
- Treatment facility
- Vitals and readings

The advanced and premium level accounts offer the highest level of access to the MyHealtheVet features. This access includes key portions of the VA health record, including:

- Admissions and discharges (including discharge summaries)
- Allergies
- Future and past appointments
- Demographic information
- Electrocardiogram
- Immunization and vaccination records
- Laboratory results
- Medication history
- Notes
- Pathology reports
- Problem list
- Radiology report
- Vitals and readings
- Wellness reminders
- Electronic health record information
- Secure messaging with providers

Regardless of the limitations or functionalities of individual systems, patients find value in an integrated patient portal system because of the convenience, the improved access, and the opportunity to take part in their own healthcare. (1)

IF YOU BUILD IT—WILL THEY COME? (5)

- Before purchasing a patient portal system, make certain it will interface with your electronic health record system; otherwise, it will be useless.
- Plan for a substantial financial investment. The costs of patient portals vary by individual EHR vendor, but this may be a factor in the low percentage of physician offices using patient portals.
- Before deciding on a particular patient portal, interview vendors and their clients. Find out how easy it is to use, ask if there are any enhancements scheduled

for the near future, find out what is required when the system is updated (downtime), or if there are routine "patches."

- Take the system for a test drive. Imagine that you are a patient and assess how easy it is to maneuver. Have other members of your staff test it—especially those who will refer your patients to the portal for information.
- Let the vendor know what your patients want and ask them to tell you whether it has already been done. If one vendor cannot provide the features that your patients need, find a vendor who will.
- Before signing a contract with a vendor, find out about vendor system support and how often this support is provided. Ask if there is a guarantee that the vendor provides to ensure the system is ready for future stages of meaningful use.
- Ensure that the vendor is willing to meet with your practice's legal team to assess security, privacy, and other legal considerations. Make certain your patients' information will be secure.
- Practices may need to implement only part of the portal first: for example, enabling patients to access for prescription refills, to request appointments, or to ask minor clinical questions. Then move to implementation of advanced functionality as staff and patients become more comfortable with the functionality of the system.
- Be ready for future applications like mobile health, telehealth, point of care, and home monitoring data that could eventually be uploaded into these portals through iPhones and other smart consumer technology.

BOTTOM LINE

Patient portals enable patients to communicate with providers, access medical records and lab test results, schedule appointments, and refill prescriptions. Portals can also increase care efficiency, improve the management of chronic illness, and actively engage patients in their own healthcare. With so many functions available and patients ready to use them, patient portals are here to stay.

Reference

1. Woodcock, EW. How Patient Portals Create Value for Patients—and Fulfill Meaningful Use Requirements, 2010. Accessed April 2014. http://www.intuithealth.com/mgma.
2. Terry, K. Patient portal explosion has major health care implications. iHealthBeat Insight, February 12, 2013. http://www.ihealthbeat.org. Accessed May 7, 2013.
3. Emont, S. Measuring the impact of patient portals: what the literature tells us. Sacramento: California Healthcare Foundation. 2011.
4. U. S. Department of Veteran Affairs. My HealtheVet account types. *https://www.myhealth. va.gov.* Accessed August 20, 2013.
5. Dolan, P. Make sure patient portals go beyond meaningful use. amednews.com, January 28, 2013. *http://amednews.com.* Accessed April 21, 2013.

CHAPTER 6

Med Rec not Med Wreck!

EDICATION RECONCILIATION (MED REC) IS the systematic and comprehensive process by which all medications a patient is currently taking are verified; doses and indications clarified; and additions, changes, and discontinuations documented in the medical record and the patient's list. Medication reconciliation can involve the provider, pharmacist, nurse, and patient, and should occur during almost all transitions of care. (1)

Medication reconciliation errors occur when there are differences among documented drug regimens, including therapeutic duplications (taking the brand name and the generic at the same time), wrong drug, wrong dose, wrong strength, omissions, drug interactions, allergies, adverse reactions, and other critical discrepancies.

Studies have shown that patients who had medication reconciliation errors after hospital admission varied from 27% to 65%. (2) At discharge, 20% to 66% of patients had one or more reconciliation errors. (3) The impact of medication reconciliation errors ranges from insignificant harm to permanent damage and even death. (2)

In 2005, the Joint Commission made medication reconciliation National Patient Safety Goal #8 (and in 2013 designated it NPSG.03.06.01). Specifically, the goal states: *Maintain and communicate accurate patient medication information. This goal has four elements of performance.*

1. Obtain information on *all* of the medication the patient is currently taking when he or she is admitted to the hospital or is seen in an outpatient setting. The information is documented in a list or other format that is useful to those who manage medications. This includes all prescription medications, over-the-counter drugs, nutritional supplements, herbal products, and anything classified by the Food and Drug Administration. The list should include the drug name, dose, frequency, and formulation.
2. Define the types of medication information to be collected in non-24-hour settings and different patient circumstances.
3. Compare the medication information the patient brought to the hospital with the medication ordered for the patient by the hospital in order to identify and resolve discrepancies.

4. Provide the patient (or family as needed) with written information on the medications the patient should be taking when he or she is discharged from the hospital or at the end of an outpatient encounter.

The Centers for Medicare and Medicaid Services also include measures related to medication reconciliation in the Core Objectives for Eligible Professionals (EP) for Stage 2 Meaningful Use and a Clinical Quality Measure (CQM) for 2014.

OBJECTIVE: The EP who receives a patient from another setting of care or provider of care or believes an encounter is relevant should perform medication reconciliation.

Stage 1 Measure and Stage 2 Measure: The EP performs medication reconciliation for more than 50% of transitions of care in which the patient is transitioned into the care of the EP.

CQM Measure: Documentation of Current Medications in the Medical Record

Description: Percentage of specified visits for patients ages 18 years and older for which the EP attests to documenting a list of current medications to the best of his or her knowledge and ability. This list must include ALL prescriptions, over-the-counters, herbals, and vitamin/mineral/dietary (nutritional) supplements, AND must include the medication's name, dosage, frequency, and route of administration.

Domain: Patient Safety

WHY MED REC IS IMPORTANT

Review and reconciliation of the patient's current medications should occur at all transfers of care in the inpatient setting. However, medication reconciliation does not apply just to the inpatient setting. Medication reconciliation should occur in the ambulatory care setting as well. It is estimated that 25% of patients have experienced an adverse drug event in the ambulatory setting. (4) Many of these events are attributed to taking medications inappropriately and could have been prevented if medication reconciliation had been performed. These errors included:

- The medication appeared active in the medical record yet the patient reported not taking it. This may be due to patient discontinuation due to an adverse reaction (fatigue, upset stomach) or allergic reaction to the drug. This may be due to the patient not having the drug prescription filled originally or not refilled due to cost. Providers may not know the patient has stopped taking the drug and, assuming therapy is ineffective, prescribe additional medication.

Medication Reconciliation Resources

The medication reconciliation initiative, MATCH, was developed through the support of the Agency for Healthcare Research and Quality (AHRQ), a collaboration between Northwestern Memorial Hospital, Northwestern University Feinberg School of Medicine, and The Joint Commission. (5)

MATCH offers a toolkit to help hospital and outpatient practice staff:

- Make the case for prioritizing medication reconciliation as a patient safety program at the organization;
- Define the problem by outlining successful practices and identifying current deficiencies within the organization or practice setting.
- Develop a new or redesign an existing medication reconciliation process that will meet patient safety goals and can be integrated into staff's workflow;
- Test and implement the new or enhanced medication reconciliation process throughout the organization or within the practice setting;
- Assess and evaluate the process post-implementation to achieve sustainable results; and
- Inform and involve patients, families, and caregivers in the medication reconciliation process.
- The materials in the toolkit can be used as guidance for developing a medication reconciliation process in your own facility.

Medications include non-opioid analgesics (tramadol, aspirin, acetaminophen), antilipemics, beta-blockers, NSAIDs, and PPIs.

- The patient reports taking one or more medications that did not appear on the active medication list. Medications include aspirin, NSAIDs, OTC proton pump inhibitors, herbal products, and nutritional supplements. In many states the legalization of marijuana has also complicated therapeutic regimens. The omission of these agents from the medication list prevents the accurate review of drug-drug interactions, allergy checks, review for therapeutic duplication, and other clinical decision support interventions.
- The patient reports taking two medications of the same therapeutic drug class at the same time. Example: anticoagulants (enoxaparin and warfarin).
- The patient reports taking the drugs, but is taking them differently than prescribed.

To reduce errors and patient harm in both the inpatient and ambulatory settings, the Agency for Healthcare Research and Quality has defined the four steps for medication reconciliation: (5)

1. **Verification.** Reviewing a patient's medication use history and developing an accurate list of all medications, including prescriptions, over-the-counter medications, vitamins, supplements, eye drops, creams, ointments, herbal products, etc., when he or she is admitted to the hospital or seen in an outpatient setting.
2. **Clarification.** Ensuring that the medications and doses are appropriate and using the current list when writing medication orders.
3. **Reconciliation.** Identifying any discrepancy between medications ordered for patients and those on the list, making appropriate changes to the orders, documenting any changes, and communicating the updated list to the next provider within or outside the hospital.
4. **Education.** Providing patients with an updated medication list and written information on the medications when discharged from the hospital.

DECREASE DISCREPANCIES

Because the majority of chronic medication prescribing occurs in the outpatient setting, providers should perform thorough and accurate medication reconciliation at each office visit. For example:

- Identify discrepancies in commission, omission, and duplication, and resolve these to improve therapeutic outcomes and reduce patient harm.
- Encourage patients to keep an accurate, up-to-date medication list with them at all times. This list can be a hard copy, flash drive, or even a list on their smart phone. The 3-ring binder, *Personal Health System* by Mary Sue McAslan is available at Amazon.com.
- Be sure that all medication allergies or adverse reactions are written on the list. Ask if there are any new allergies or adverse reactions.
- At each visit, ask if any new medications are being taken. Who prescribed them and why?
- Ask if the patient has stopped taking any medication and why.
- Ask if there are any medications that the patient is not taking as originally prescribed and why. This may lead to a discussion of adverse reactions or side effects, which can be avoided with specific instructions such as taking with food to avoid GI upset or taking at bedtime to avoid drowsiness.
- If patients are not taking a medication as prescribed or have stopped taking a medication altogether due to cost, there are several options to pursue. Generic substitution or therapeutic substitution may work well. Have patients ask the pharmacist for recommendations before filling the prescription.
- Pay attention to early refills. This may be a warning that the medication is not working as prescribed or that patient is taking it inappropriately.

Over-the-counter medication, herbal products, supplements, and marijuana can all lead to significant patient harm. Be sure that patients list all of these products on their med list and that these are discussed as part of the medication reconciliation process.

BOTTOM LINE

Medication discrepancies can cause serious medication errors. Medication reconciliation is intended to identify and resolve these discrepancies and prevent these errors before they occur.

References

1. Greenwald, JL. Making inpatient medication reconciliation patient-centered, clinically relevant, and implementable: A consensus statement on key principles and necessary first steps. *J Hosp Med*. 2010 Oct; 5(8):477-485. doi: 10.1002/jhm.849.
2. Tam, VC, et al. Frequency, type and clinical importance of medication history errors at admission to hospital: A systematic review. *CMAJ*. 2005 Aug 30; 173(5):510-515.
3. Forster AJ, Clark HD, Menard A, et al. Adverse events among medical patients after discharge from hospital. *CMAJ*. 2004 Feb 3;170 (3):345-349.
4. Gandhi TK, Weingart SN, Borus J, et al. Adverse drug events in ambulatory care. *N Engl J Med*. 2003 Apr 17; 348(16):1556-1564.
5. Gleason KM, McDaniel MR, Feinglass J, et al. Results of the medications at transitions and clinical handoffs (MATCH) study: An analysis of medication reconciliation errors and risk factors at hospital admission. *J Gen Intern Med*. 2010 May; 25(5):441-447. doi: 10.1007/s11606-010-1256-6.

CHAPTER 7

Back to Basics: The Med List

A S A PHARMACIST, I KNOW FIRST-HAND the importance of knowing *all* of the medications that a patient is or is not taking. During the hospital admission, transfer, and discharge process, as well as the ambulatory care process, a thorough and accurate reconciliation of each medication the patient is taking with the list in the medical record should be performed to ensure providers are aware of any serious and harmful discrepancies.

Accurate medication reconciliation (and the subsequent identification of serious medication discrepancies) depends on the patient maintaining an up-to-date medication record. This record can be a hardcopy, a flash drive, or even a list on their smart phone. Whatever the format, this list should include all of the prescription drugs prescribed by all providers, as well as over-the-counter drugs (pain relievers, acid blockers, antihistamines, sedatives, weight loss agents, etc.) vitamins, nutritional supplements, herbal products, eye drops, creams, ointments, nasal sprays, etc. In states where medical marijuana is legal, this should be included on the list as well.

The med list should include the name of the drug, the name of the doctor who prescribed it and when, the dose, how often the patient is taking it, and why it was prescribed. The list should include the date the drug was started and stopped, if applicable, and the reason it was stopped. The list must include any medication allergies, food allergies, or allergies to other products such as latex. Patients should also include any adverse reactions or side effects to drugs that have occurred in the past, such as myalgia to statins or cough due to an ACE inhibitor.

The medication list is critical to help ensure patient safety during any inpatient transition of care or ambulatory care visit. Having an accurate record of what the patient is taking can help prevent serious errors such as omissions, therapeutic duplications, or prescription of a drug that the patient is allergic to.

WHY IT'S IMPORTANT

- Quickly and concisely provides the clinician with a list of prescription medications that the patient is actually taking (or not taking), including those prescribed by other doctors.

- Provides the clinician with a list of over-the-counter agents the patient is taking.
- Provides the clinician with knowledge of other substances the patient is using, such as marijuana.
- Identifies and reduces the opportunity for medication discrepancies, including duplications, omissions, or interactions.
- Supports medication reconciliation process.
- Reinforces with the patient the names of medications, why they are used, how they should be taken, and what side effects to watch for.
- Reduces medication errors in a simple and cost-effective manner.
- Encourages physician communication with patients for safer healthcare.

WHAT THE PROVIDER CAN DO

- Provide patients with a blank copy of a medication list and ask them to fill it out before they come in for their office visit. Medications on the patient's list should include all prescription drugs, over-the-counter agents (antihistamines, proton-pump inhibitors for GERD, NSAIDs etc.), vitamins and supplements, herbal products, and natural remedies. This list also needs to include marijuana if applicable, as this is now legal in some states.
- If the patient does not carry a medication list, obtain medication information from the family member or caregiver if possible.
- Compare the medications the patient is currently taking to medications being prescribed for the patient and identify and resolve discrepancies.
- Provide the patient or caregiver with an up-to-date list of all medications the patient should be taking and instructions about how he or she should be taking them before the patient leaves the office or hospital setting.
- Make sure the patient understands how to take these medications before he or she leaves the office or hospital.
- Provide the patient with resources that will help him or her take the medications appropriately. These resources may help overcome language and health literacy barriers.
- Ask the patient to take a copy of the list to any other provider visits he or she may have, and review the list with all providers, including dentists, therapists, pharmacists, nutritionists, etc.
- Tell the patient to review the list with his or her pharmacist and to obtain any information necessary to take the medications correctly, including allergies, drug-drug interactions, drug-OTC interactions, drug-food interactions, drug-alcohol interactions, drug-herbal interactions, etc.
- Instruct patients to contact their providers or pharmacist whenever there is a question about their medications (before they take the drug).

BOTTOM LINE

Patients should create a medication list and keep it with them at all times. The medication list is one of the most important things patients can do to prevent serious errors leading to hospital admissions or readmissions.

How to Create a Simple Medication List

Patients can make their own medication list by using the form provided here or by going to www.drmarysue.com to download a free copy. By following the steps below, patients can quickly create a complete medication list.

☐ Line up all prescription bottles and over-the-counter medications on the table in front of you. Include vitamins, herbal products, nutritional supplements, and all other meds, as well as creams and ointments, patches, eye drops, eardrops, and nose drops or sprays. Include medical marijuana. Be sure to list medications that you take routinely as well as medications you take only occasionally.

☐ For each medication, read the label and fill in the information from the label on the medication list. Include the date you started taking the drug, the name of the drug, what it's for, how you take it, and any known side effects.

☐ Update the list when dosages change or when you stop or start a new medication.

☐ Always keep the med list with you. Fold it and keep it in your wallet or purse.

☐ Be sure to give a copy to your spouse, partner, children, and other caregivers.

☐ Take the list with you to all healthcare appointments, including those with doctors, dentists, therapists, and others. Doctors are now asking their patients to bring an updated med list with them to their appointments. Having it filled out beforehand can save time for you and your doctor and prevent errors.

☐ Review the list with your doctor at each office visit to ensure that the doctor's list matches yours and that you are taking your medications as prescribed.

☐ If your medication list does not match the doctor's list, clear up any differences with your doctor during the office visit (before you go home).

☐ Bring a copy of the list to the pharmacy when you have your prescriptions filled and have the pharmacist review it to make sure your list matches the pharmacy's records.

☐ If you have new allergies, update your doctor and pharmacist with new allergy information.

☐ If you have questions about filling out the medication list, ask your pharmacist for help.

☐ You can keep a medication list in many possible formats, including a piece of paper, portable flash drive, software application for your computer, or app for your smart phone; however, many hospitals and doctor's offices do not accept these drives into their computer systems because of privacy issues and concern about computer viruses.

☐ Keep both a paper copy of your medication list and an electronic copy and update both as often as necessary.

Medication List

Name: _____   Date: _____

Medication Allergies or Reactions: _____

Name of Pharmacy: _____

Phone Number of Pharmacy: _____

Start Date	Name/strength of medicine*	How I take medicine	Reason I take medicine	Doctor	Stop Date

*Include all vitamins, herbal supplements, nutritional products, antacids, laxatives, allergy relief products, and other over-the-counter medications.

CHAPTER 8

Improving the Quality of Care

CLINICAL QUALITY MEASURES (CQMs) ARE tools that help measure and track the quality of healthcare services provided by eligible professionals (EPs) in our healthcare systems. (1) Using a wide range of data, CQMs provide information on health outcomes, clinical processes, patient safety, efficient use of health resources, care coordination, patient engagements, population, and public health and clinical guidelines. (1) By continuously monitoring these measures, we can help ensure the sustainability of safe, high-quality patient care.

RECOMMENDED CORE SETS

In Stage 1 Meaningful Use, CQM reporting was required as a core objective. In Stage 2, CQMs are no longer a core objective; however, all providers are required to report on CQMs in order to demonstrate meaningful use. Beginning in 2014, all providers regardless of their stage of meaningful use will report on CQMs in the same way. There are two recommended core sets of CQMs: one for adults and one for children. EPs are encouraged to report from the recommended core set to the extent that those CQMs pertain to their scope of practice and patient population. (2)

Adult Recommended Core Measures

- Controlling High Blood Pressure
- Use of High Risk Medications in the Elderly
- Preventive Care and Screening: Tobacco Use Screening and Cessation Intervention
- Use of Imaging Studies for Low Back Pain
- Preventive Care and Screening: Screening for Clinical Depression and Follow-Up Plan
- Documentation of Current Medications in the Medical Record
- Preventive Care and Screening: Body Mass Index (BMI) Screening and Follow-Up
- Closing the Referral Loop: Receipt of Specialist Report

Pediatric Recommended Core Measures

- Appropriate Testing for Children with Pharyngitis
- Weight Assessment and Counseling for Nutrition and Physical Activity for Children and Adolescents
- Chlamydia Screening for Women
- Use of Appropriate Medications for Asthma
- Childhood Immunization Status
- Appropriate Treatment for Children with Upper Respiratory Infection (URI)
- ADHD: Follow-Up Care for Children Prescribed Attention-Deficit/Hyperactivity Disorder (ADHD) Medication
- Preventive Care and Screening: Screening for Clinical Depression and Follow-Up Plan
- Dental Decay or Cavities

2014 CQM REPORTING OPTIONS

In 2014, electronic health record technology will include new CQM criteria and EPs will begin reporting using the new 2014 criteria regardless of whether they are participating in Stage 1 or Stage 2 of the Medicare and Medicaid Electronic Health Record Incentive Programs. (3)

EPs will report on 9 of the 64 approved CQMs:

- Recommended core CQMs (encouraged but not required).
- 9 CQMs for the adult population.
- 9 CQMs for the pediatric population.
- NQF 0018 strongly encouraged because controlling blood pressure is a high priority goal in national health initiatives, including the Million Hearts campaign.

In addition, providers must select CQMs from at least three of the six healthcare policy domains recommended by the Department of Health and Human Services National Quality Strategy:

1. Patient and Family Engagement
2. Patient Safety
3. Care Coordination
4. Population and Public Health
5. Efficient Use of Healthcare Resources
6. Clinical Processes/Effectiveness

ECQMS

In 2014, all Medicare-eligible providers beyond their first year of demonstrating meaningful use must electronically report their CQM data to the Centers for Medicare and Medicaid (CMS). EPs can report using the Physician Quality

Reporting System (PQRS) or the CMS-designated transmission method. For 2014 only, all providers regardless of their stage of meaningful use, are only required to demonstrate meaningful use for a three-month EHR reporting period. This three-month reporting period is permitted so that all providers who must upgrade to the 2014 certified technology have adequate time to do so. In subsequent years, the reporting for CQMs will be the entire calendar year.

Despite the three-month reporting provision, the electronic reporting of clinical quality measures may be easier said than done. Hospitals are reporting that it is harder to use their EHRs to report eCQMs than they expected. (4) They are reporting unanticipated increased costs and the unplanned need to modify data captures to meet eCQM tool requirements. Vendors delivered eCQM specifications that had errors, or the eCQM tools did not produce accurate measures. Finally, but most importantly, the eCQMS added to physicians' workloads and provided no perceived benefit to patient care. (4)

WHAT'S THE RUSH?

In an effort to improve the *quality of reporting* of the clinical quality measures, the American Hospital Association recommended that the government slow the pace of requiring CQMs. (5) AHA also recommended the use of fewer but better-tested CQMs and improved measuring tools. They recommended that users be provided with clear guidance and a consistent process, and that the program support accurate measurement. (5) The fear among many hospitals and providers is that with the rapid "all-or-nothing" implementation of new requirements and the mandated 2014 electronic reporting procedures, they will not be able to meet the requirements of meaningful use and not qualify for the Medicaid and Medicare incentive payments.

CQMS—A WORK IN PROGRESS

- Be sure to select CQMs from at least three of the six healthcare policy domains.
- When selecting CQMs for your practice, select those that closely align with your patient population. If one of the adult or pediatric recommended core measures does not pertain to your patients, select one from the other 64 measures that does.
- Use EHR technology to identify patient-specific clinical reminders for preventive care and screening. This will help ensure adherence with CQM screening requirements for tobacco use, clinical depression, and body mass index.
- Ask your EHR vendor if the system will support the 2014 reporting requirements and if not, what they will do to upgrade it.

- Work with vendors before, during, and after upgrades. Vendors need time to develop and test upgrades and providers need time to implement them and maximize their use before another upgrade comes along.

BOTTOM LINE

Reporting clinical quality measures is a great way to track the implementation and ensure the sustainability of quality improvement efforts; however, these measures represent tremendous changes in practice in many institutions. These are clinical quality improvement changes that take a great deal of time to implement and cannot be forced. The infrastructure to support these changes, both in the actual clinical quality improvement effort and the technological systems to measure it, must be firmly in place before any effort is undertaken or it will be doomed to fail.

References

1. Centers for Medicare and Medicaid Services. Clinical quality measures (CQMs). Centers for Medicare and Medicaid Services. *http://www.cms.gov*. Accessed August 21, 2013.
2. Centers for Medicare and Medicaid Services. Recommended core measures. Centers for Medicare and Medicaid Services. *http://www.cms.gov*. Accessed August 21, 2013.
3. Centers for Medicare and Medicaid Services. 2014 clinical quality measures tipsheet. Centers for Medicare and Medicaid Services. *http://www.cms.gov*. Accessed August 21, 2013.
4. Monegain B. AHA urges quality reporting slowdown. *Healthcare IT News*. *http://www.health-careitnews.com*. Accessed August 21, 2013.
5. Hirsch MD. 5 recommendations for generating electronic clinical quality measures. FierceEMR. *http://www.fierceemr.com*. Accessed August 21, 2013.

CHAPTER 9

Summaries and Transitions of Care

P ROVIDING A PATIENT'S SUMMARY OF CARE to another provider is essential to ensuring high-quality, coordinated healthcare. A summary of care record helps ensure accurate and complete communication of critical information, helps decrease the need for and costs associated with repeated tests, and provides timely transmission of information necessary to initiate new or emergent treatment. The summary of care record includes at a minimum: (1)

- Patient name;
- Referring or transitioning provider's name and office contact information (EP only);
- Procedures;
- Encounter diagnosis;
- Immunizations;
- Laboratory test results;
- Vital signs (height, weight, blood pressure, BMI);
- Smoking status;
- Functional status, including activities of daily living, cognitive and disability status;
- Demographic information (preferred language, sex, race, ethnicity, date of birth);
- Care plan field, including goals and instructions;
- Care team, including the primary care provider of record and any additional known care team members beyond the referring or transitions provider and the receiving provider;
- Reason for referral;
- Current problem list (EPs may also include historical problems at their discretion);
- Current medication list; and
- Current medication allergy list.

Summaries of care are important in helping providers make timely and well-informed decisions based on up-to-date health data. If provided electronically, summaries of care can be incorporated directly into the receiving provider's electronic health records. They reduce the need for the patient to transport paper copies of records and help with the registration process by decreasing the need for patients to complete forms during the first visit.

In Stage 2 Meaningful Use, the Centers for Medicare and Medicaid Services (CMS) changed the Transitions of Care objective in Stage 1 by moving it from the menu set into the core objectives and increasing the number of measures from one to three. Many providers are concerned about how they will successfully meet all of the requirements of this complex, yet critical measure.

The objective for the Stage 2 Meaningful Use Transition of Care Summary states that "the EP who transitions their patient to another setting of care or provider of care or refers their patient to another provider of care should provide a summary of care record for each transition of care or referral."

STAGE 2 MEASURES

1. The EP who transitions or refers a patient to another setting of care provides a summary of care record for more than 50% of transitions of care and referrals.
2. The EP who transitions or refers a patient to another setting of care or provider of care provides a summary of care record either a) electronically transmitted to a recipient using certified electronic health record technology or b) where the recipient receives the summary of care record via exchange facilitated by an organization that is a eHealth Exchange participant or is validated through an ONC-established governance mechanism to facilitate exchange for 10% of transitions and referrals.
3. The EP who transitions or refers a patient to another setting of care or provider of care must either a) conduct one or more successful electronic exchanges of a summary of care record with a recipient using technology that was designed by a different EHR developer than the sender's, or b) conduct one or more successful tests with the CMS-designated test EHR during the EHR reporting period.

Transitions of care are defined as the movement of a patient from one setting of care (hospital, ambulatory primary care practice, ambulatory specialty care practice, long-term care, home health, rehabilitation facility) to another. (1) To meet this definition, there must be a provider recipient. As a result, CMS states that "a transition home without any expectation of follow-up care related to the care given in the prior setting by another provider is not a transition of care for purposes of Stage 2 Meaningful Use measures." In addition, a transition within the hospital or a setting of care does not qualify as a transition of care.

The certified EHR technology has the capability to calculate the data for this measure. The denominator includes the number of transitions of care and referrals during the reporting period and the numerator is the number of transitions of care and referrals in the denominator where a summary of care record was provided.

THIS IS NOT GOING TO BE EASY.....

- Providers who are not employed by a hospital or large integrated health system will certainly find it difficult to meet this standard. These physicians and practices will need to build their own networks with providers they refer patients to and hospitals they admit patients to. Additionally, these providers will incur a cost for participating in local health information exchanges and need to pay the EHR vendors added fees to support required protocols.
- Providers should work with EHR vendors to test and certify to particular transmission standards. Providers may use an intermediary such as a Health Information Exchange (HIE) or Health Information Service Providers (HISP) to facilitate the exchange of the summary of care record.
- A certified electronic health record must be able to electronically receive and display a patient's summary of care record from other providers and organizations, including at a minimum, diagnostic test results, problem list, medication list, and medication allergy list, and enable a user to electronically transmit a patient summary record to other providers and organizations.
- CMS prefers that the summary of care record is generated electronically, but acknowledges that the EP or hospital may need to send a hard copy to the next provider. However, a certified EHR system must be used to *generate* the summary of care record and document whether it was given directly to the provider or given to the patient to deliver to the provider.
- CMS states "to count in the numerator, the summary of care record must be received by the provider to whom the sending provider is referring or transferring the patient." If the summary is sent directly to the receiving provider, then the CEHRT can count these transactions in the numerator. However, if the summary is sent to the HIE or HISP and you rely on the receiving provider to pull the document, you must have validation that the summary was retrieved for it to count.
- If the provider to whom the referral is made has access to the medical record maintained by the referring provider, then the summary of care record does not need to be provided. This may be the case in managed care organizations or other large, integrated healthcare systems.

BOTTOM LINE

Providing a summary of a patient's healthcare data to another provider is critical to ensuring the coordination of care. However, meeting the measures of Stage 2 Meaningful Use Transition of Care summary may prove to be a daunting task.

Working with EHR vendors to optimize current systems and build an operational roadmap to implement over the next few years will help meet these challenging standards.

Reference

1. Centers for Medicare and Medicaid Services. Stage 2eligible professional meaningful use core measures. Centers for Medicare and Medicaid Services. *http://www.cms.gov*. Accessed August 15, 2013.

CHAPTER 10

Meeting the MU Challenge

THE TRANSITION FROM Stage 1 Meaningful Use to Stage 2 Meaningful Use has presented an unexpected challenge for some eligible professionals (EPs) and hospitals. Stage 2 Meaningful Use represents an expanded and more consistent level of adherence and reporting. In Stage 1, providers had to prove they were capable of performing certain objectives with electronic health record systems. In Stage 2, practices will be required to demonstrate performance with these objectives as well as other more rigorous objectives. Hospitals and EPs who complied with Stage 1 must be aware that reporting percentages have increased in Stage 2, the number of clinical quality measures has increased, there are new requirements regarding patient engagement, and a fewer number of measures can be excluded. Providers should be aware of these high- impact changes and plan to implement strategies to address them.

WHAT CONCERNS YOU THE MOST?

There are three measures in Stage 2 Meaningful Use that may present a challenge to practices and hospitals:

1. **Patient Engagement:** In Stage 1 Meaningful Use, practices were required to provide patients with an electronic copy of their health information upon request. The measure required that more than 50% of all patients who requested an electronic copy were provided it within three business days. For the most part, this did not create too much of a problem; many providers did not advertise this to their patients so few people requested their health information.

   In Stage 2, practices must provide patients the ability to view online, download, and transmit their health information within four business days of the information being available to the EP. The first measure requires that more than 50% of patients are provided timely online access to their health information; however, the second measure requires that *more than 5% of all patients seen by the EP during the reporting period, view, download, or transmit to a third party their health information.* While 5% may seem like a low threshold for this measure, it still means that practices will need to implement systems such as patient portals to ensure access to health information.

Patient portals are costly and staff members will need to be trained in their use and then, in turn, they must train patients in how to use them. Even then, there is no guarantee that patients will actually go into the portal and view their records.

2. **Summaries of Care:** In Stage 2 Meaningful Use, the EP who transitions or refers a patient to another provider or setting of care, provides a summary of care record for more than 50% of these transitions or referrals. The first measure requires that in 10% of those transitions, the summary must be transmitted electronically using a 2014 edition of certified EHR. This summary will need to be in a specific format known as the consolidated CDA (C-CDA) rather than the Continuity of Care Document (CCD) or Continuity of Care Record (CCR).

   Neither the CCD nor the CCR include the required data elements necessary to meet the summary of care objective. Providers must ensure that they are using the correct EHR edition: Transitions of Care—Create and Transmit Transition of Care/Referral Summaries.

3. **Clinical Quality Measures:** In Stage 1 Meaningful Use, practices were required to report clinical quality measures (CQMs) to CMS or to the states. The Stage 1 measure was to provide aggregate numerator, denominator, and exclusions through attestation or through the PQRS electronic reporting pilot. In Stage 2, this measure has been removed; instead, CMS proposed recommended core measures aligned with high priority healthcare improvement goals.

   Beginning in 2014, all providers must report 9 CQMs (up from 6 CQMs) and hospitals must report 16 (up from 15 CQMs). Providers, beyond their first year of participation, must report data to CMS electronically. In essence, Stage 2 Meaningful Use emphasizes the importance of reporting clinical quality measures. Providers will need to identify the CQMs that closely align with their practices and patient populations and work with EHR vendors to build systems capable of data extraction and accurate reporting mechanisms.

   At the time of this writing, the American Hospital Association has called for a delay in the deadline for Stage 2 Meaningful Use for the clinical quality measures. (1) It cites the need for fewer, better-tested measures, with reporting tools that are more flexible and interoperable. It also calls for an improvement in testing eCQMs for reliability and validity before adopting them in national programs.

   Lastly, it is asking for clear guidance and tested tools to support hospital transition to electronic reporting requirements. Whatever the outcome of this request, providers will need to select their CQMs wisely and prepare and strategize with their EHR vendors to ensure accurate and complete reporting.

PREVENTING THE PITFALLS OF STAGE 2 MEANINGFUL USE

- Providers in small practices and large healthcare institutions who do not understand the requirements for demonstrating meaningful use should research questions online at *www.cms.gov.*
- Be sure you have the 2014 edition of certified EHR technology and that your hardware and software can support the reporting requirements. This is especially important for the new summaries of care data sets as well as the clinical quality measures.
- Be sure to review all exclusions. Providers may decide not to pursue meaningful use if they see a core measure that they feel they cannot meet. However, many of these core measures have exclusions that should be evaluated before giving up. (2)
- Be proactive when dealing with EHR vendors. Do not delay implementation until it is too late to accurately process and report measurement data.
- Allow time to train staff and let them adjust to new procedures. This includes the transition from paper to electronic health records; e-prescribing; and recording, organizing, and retrieving data electronically.
- Be sure you know who should have access and that you control access to patient health information. Ensure that data is properly encrypted and that it is stored properly to prevent breaches in confidentiality.
- Run meaningful use reports routinely and frequently. If possible, schedule these reports to run automatically so you can review, analyze and fix any problems before your percentages start to drop.

BOTTOM LINE

Reporting core objectives and clinical quality measures for eligible professionals and hospitals will take a real team effort. Including the EHR vendor, all healthcare providers, the practice staff, and patients will help to ensure the successful reporting of the quality measures and also help provide coordinated, high-quality healthcare.

References

1. Commins J. Citing 'system failure' AHA urges delay of meaningful use stage 2. Health Leaders Media. http://www.healthleadersmedia.com/content/tec-294674/citing-system-failure-aha-urges-delay-of-mu-stage-2. Accessed September 14, 2013.
2. Vacca K. The 7 deadly sins of meaningful use—and how to avoid them. PhysBiz Tech. *http://www.physbiztech.com/print/4441.* Accessed September 14, 2013.

Reduce Readmissions

"Nothing about me without me."

VALERIE BILLINGHAM

CHAPTER 11

Person-Centered Care

PERSON-CENTERED CARE (also known as patient-centered care or PCC) is a complex and multi-dimensional concept that is increasingly recognized as the optimal form of care in all types of healthcare venues, including primary, acute, and long-term settings. (1) In 2001, the Institute of Medicine (IOM) identified person-centered care as one of the six determinants of high-quality care.

The IOM defines person-centered care as healthcare that establishes a partnership among practitioners, patients, and their families (when appropriate) to ensure that decisions respect patients' wants, needs, and preferences, and that patients have the education and support they need to make decisions and participate in their own care.

Recent evidence has shown that adoption of patient-centered care has led to improved outcomes, including reduced lengths of stay, avoided readmissions and emergency department visits, and increased patient satisfaction and employee engagement. (2) The Centers for Medicare and Medicaid (CMS) has made patient-centered care and the patient experience a priority by using the patient perception of care (through the HCAHPS) a part of the value-based purchasing calculation influencing hospitals' CMS reimbursement. This policy change has elevated patient-centered care from a "feel-good" concept to a financial imperative. (3)

THE PLANETREE MODEL

The Planetree model of patient-centered care was created in 1978. The Planetree philosophy states that care should be organized first and foremost around the needs of the patient. However, achieving the tenets of this philosophy requires more than just a quick training course and a change in operations; it requires a complete cultural transformation from one that is disease-centered or problem-based to being person-centered and wellness-based. This shift requires a major change in operations, strategic planning, resources, and provision of care. (4)

Although no magic bullet exists for the implementation of PCC, Planetree endorses 10 components that create a customizable framework for the development of patient-centered care. (5) These include:

1. **Human Interactions**—Creating organizational cultures that support caring, kindness, and respect in all interactions between patients, families, and staff members.

2. **Family, Friends, and Social Support**—Encouraging the involvement of family and friends as partners in the care experience, whenever possible, offering patient-directed visitation, including in the ICU and ED, family presence protocols, and care partner programs.

3. **Access to Information**—Providing patients with information and educational resources so they can actively participate in their own care. Patients have access to their medical charts, can take part in collaborative care conferences (in which the patient, family, physician, and nurse converse at the bedside), and can visit libraries or Planetree Health Resource Centers that are open to the community and offer health and medical information.

4. **Healing Environments Through Architectural Design**—Creating quiet, healing environments using evidence-based design principles that create homelike and welcoming settings that remove barriers between patients, families, and caregivers.

5. **Food and Nutrition**—Providing delicious, healthful meals and making good food choices available to patients, families, and staff 24 hours a day, seven days a week.

6. **Arts and Entertainment**—Creating an atmosphere of serenity and playfulness by displaying artwork in the patient rooms and treatment areas, having volunteers work with patients to create their own art, and inviting local artists and musicians to help lift spirits by exposing patients to the arts and entertainment.

7. **Spirituality**—Helping patients, families, and staff connect with their own inner resources by providing access to clergy and places of worship, gardens, labyrinths, and meditation rooms.

8. **Human Touch**—Using caring touch and massage to reduce anxiety, pain, and stress in patients, families, and staff members.

9. **Therapies**—Expanding choice by offering patients access or referral to aromatherapy, Reiki, guided imagery, therapeutic touch, acupuncture, chiropractic, Tai Chi, yoga, and other integrative modalities.

10. **Healthy Communities**—Increasing the role of hospitals and redefining healthcare to include the health and wellness of the community by working with schools, senior citizen centers, churches, and other community partners.

Adopting patient-centered care—whether it is Planetree or another methodology—with the resultant expectation that there will be a cultural change, requires extensive commitment from medical staff and senior leaders. This commitment needs to be fully embraced by nurse managers and department managers to ensure that front-line staff knows this is not just another "flavor of the month" QI program, but a complete change in operations.

CREATING CULTURAL CHANGE

- Patient-centered care (PCC) requires extensive employee training and an "adaptive reserve" of time and resources. Institutions that do not anticipate the lengthy and costly process of cultural change may be doomed to fail.
- Keep the tenets of patient-centered care visible and vocal. Communicate frequently any new changes that are the result of these activities.
- To ensure sustainability of PCC programs, build these into the daily operations of the facility. If nutritious meals, available 24/7, are part of the model, then systems need to be firmly in place to support this.
- Changing the culture of an organization is not like reversing the course of a battleship, it is like changing the direction of the Golden Gate Bridge. Take it slow and expect delays and roadblocks.
- It is advisable to initiate cultural changes that coincide with facility architectural changes to provide tangible evidence of change. If you begin the PCC training too far ahead of physical change, employees will forget what patient-centered care is.
- Facilities may wish to initiate patient-centeredness by focusing on the wellness of their employees first. One facility started an employee fun and fitness committee, using the skills of employees to teach yoga, Tai Chi, and aerobics. Programs were taught during lunch hour and after work. One drawback was that frontline staff members were unable to attend these sessions due to workload. Ask managers to relieve staff for these classes. This builds camaraderie and morale.
- Use pet therapy when possible. This is great for patients and families. One facility used the daily walk of the rehab golden retriever as a lunchtime group fitness walk in a nearby park.
- Expand communication with employees by using emails, newsletters, social media, blogs, and other resources where appropriate. Keep up-to-date email and phone lists.
- Ask hospital volunteers, employees, residents, and patients to help plant gardens and other outdoor meditative areas.
- Ask hospital volunteers, employees, residents, and patients to bring an instrument to play for patients and families.
- Ask hospital volunteers, employees, residents, and patients to paint pictures to hang in the patient and resident areas. One hospital asked an employee to paint a mural on the back stairway. This transformed a plain white wall into a beautiful, three-story landscape!

BOTTOM LINE

Creating and sustaining a cultural change in a healthcare organization takes time, resources, dedication, and perseverance. Ensuring there is a comprehensive framework for action and an "adaptive reserve" of resources will help create and sustain this change in your organization.

References

1. Berwick, DM. What 'patient-centered' should mean: Confessions of an extremist. *Health Aff.* 2009 July/August; 28(40): w555–w565.

2. Jarousse, L. Putting patients first. *Trustee.* 2011 November/December.

3. Shaw G. The new patient experience imperative. Healthleaders Media. http://content.hcpro.com/pdf/content/269673.pdf. August 2011.

4. Guastello S, Lepore M. *Advancing PCC across the continuum of care.* Derby, CT: Planetree, 2012.

5. Planetree. About us. Planetree. http://planetree.org/about-planetree. Accessed January 26, 2013.

CHAPTER 12

Collaborate, Coordinate, and Integrate

MEASURES OF "QUALITY" have always been limited to disease-specific indicators such as beta-blocker post MI, LDL targets, HbA1c goals, and blood pressure control. Though these clinical measures appeared to be appropriate for many patients, they often missed the point for those with advanced illnesses, severe disability, and multiple co-morbidities. For those patients, "quality of care" meant more than reaching arbitrary targets, it meant an improved quality of life evidenced by improved physical status, increased mobility, reduced pain, and engagement in social functions. (1) Consideration of the patient's personal goals and preferences is the key to providing patient-centered care.

The Institute of Medicine (IOM) defines patient-centered care as "care that is respectful of and responsive to individual patient preferences, needs and values" and that ensures "that patient values guide all clinical decisions." In research prepared by the Picker Institute, it was found that eight characteristics were the most important indicators of quality and safety from the patient's perspective. (2) These are:

1. Respect for the patient's values, preferences and expressed needs;
2. Coordinated and integrated care;
3. Clear, high-quality information and education for the patient and family;
4. Physical comfort, including pain management;
5. Emotional support and alleviation of fear and anxiety;
6. Involvement of family members and friends, as appropriate;
7. Continuity, including through care-site transitions; and
8. Access to care.

Shifting from disease-specific measures to patient-centered outcomes will require a change in approach, including collaboration between the provider, patient, caregiver, and family. This collaborative approach is the fundamental concept and one of the most important strategies for improving the quality of care. To facilitate the transition to patient-centered care, the Centers for Medicare and Medicaid Services has established the Partnership for Patients with over 3,700 participating hospitals focused on making hospital care safer, more reliable, and less costly.

PARTNERSHIP FOR PATIENTS

The Partnership for Patients initiative is a public-private partnership working to improve the quality, safety, and affordability of healthcare for all Americans. (3)

The partnership is formed of physicians, nurses, hospitals, employers, patients and their advocates, and the federal and state governments.

The goals of the Partnership for Patients are to make care safer and to improve care transitions.

1. Making Care Safer—In a recent study by the Office of the Inspector General (OIG) it was found that 13% of hospitalized Medicare beneficiaries experienced adverse events resulting in a prolonged hospital stay, *permanent harm, life-sustaining intervention, or death. Almost half of those events were considered preventable.*

Goal: By the end of 2013, preventable hospital-acquired conditions would decrease by 40% compared to 2010.

There are 10 areas of focus in making care safer:

- Adverse drug events;
- Catheter-associated urinary tract infections;
- Central line associated blood stream infections;
- Injuries from falls and immobility;
- Obstetrical adverse events;
- Pressure ulcers;
- Surgical site infections;
- Venous thromboembolism;
- Ventilator-associated pneumonia; and
- Readmissions.

2. Improving Care Transitions—Care transitions are the movement of patients from one healthcare provider or setting to another. For persons living with chronic illness, transitions in care are highly prone to adverse events. An adverse event is an injury resulting from medical management rather than the underlying disease. It is estimated that one in five patients discharged from the hospital to home experience an adverse event within three weeks of discharge. The most common adverse events are medication events which can often be mitigated or completely prevented.

Goal: By the end of 2013, preventable complications during transition from one care setting to another would be decreased so that all hospital readmissions would be reduced by 20% compared to 2010.

The Partnership for Patients is composed of three key elements.

1. Hospital Engagement Networks

There are 26 Hospital Engagement Networks (HENs) across the country. These HENs are made up of state, regional, national, and hospital system organizations that help identify effective solutions and disseminate them to other hospitals and providers.

The areas of focus of Hospital Engagement Networks are: (3)

- Developing learning collaboratives for hospitals;
- Providing a wide array of initiatives and activities to improve patient safety;
- Conducting intensive training programs to help hospitals make patient care safer;
- Providing technical assistance to help hospitals achieve quality measurement goals;
- Establishing and implementing systems to track and monitor hospital progress in meeting quality improvement goals; and
- Identifying high performing hospitals and their leaders to coach and serve as national faculty to other hospitals committed to achieving the Partnership goals.

2. The Community-Based Care Transitions Program

Transitions in care happen when a patient moves from one healthcare provider or setting to another. It is estimated that one in five Medicare patients discharged from the hospital—approximately 2.6 million seniors—is readmitted within 30 days at a cost of over $26 billion every year. (3) Hospitals provide discharge planning but there is clearly a gap in care when the patient gets home. The Community-Based Care Transitions Program (CCTP) aims to create collaboration among community providers to improve the quality of care, reduce readmissions, reduce cost, and improve the patient experience.

Forty-seven sites are currently participating in the Community-Based Care Transitions Program. Each site represents a combined community effort made up of social services, Area Agencies on Aging, hospital partners, nursing homes, home health agencies, pharmacies, primary care providers, and other community healthcare partners. These CCTP sites focus on improving care transitions from the hospital to other settings for high-risk Medicare beneficiaries.

3. Patient and Family Engagement

The collaboration between healthcare providers and their patients is key to improved transitions and reduced readmissions. (3) Hospitals across the country are working diligently to advance patient and family engagement. The goal of the Partnership is to leverage existing networks, tools, and resources to promote common patient safety goals. The Partnership for Patients is working to identify and distribute patient and family engagement best practices to over 3,700 member hospitals in the Hospital Engagement Network.

APPROACHES TO COLLABORATIVE CARE

- Patients should be informed, educated, and encouraged to play a role in the decisions about their own healthcare.
- Physicians, office staff, and other healthcare professionals should provide the necessary tools and resources that patients will need to make informed choices.
- Collaboration or shared-decision making can make patients aware of the options available to them, including professional organizations and community agencies, and the importance of their preferences in the decision-making process.
- Patients should receive psychological support to enable them to voice their concerns, values and preferences and to ask questions without judgment. (4)
- Providers should ask, "What matters to you?" rather than "What is the matter?" (4)

BOTTOM LINE

Collaboration between hospitals, community programs, and the patient themselves will help achieve the two goals of improving care transitions and making hospital care safer.

References

1. Reuben DB, Tinetti ME. Goal-oriented patient care—an alternative health outcomes paradigm. *N Engl J Med.* 2012 Mar 1;366(9):777–779. doi: 10.1056/NEJMp1113631.
2. Gerteis M, Edgman-Levitan S, Daley J, Delbanco, T. *Through the Patient's Eyes.* San Franciso: Jossey Bass, 1993.
3. Centers for Medicare and Medicaid Services. Partnership for patients. Centers for Medicare and Medicaid Services. http://innovation.cms.gov/. Accessed April 22, 2013.
4. Barry MJ, Edgman-Levitan S. Shared decision making—pinnacle of patient-centered care. *N Engl J Med.* 2012 Mar 1;366(9):780–781. doi: 10.1056/NEJMp1109283.

CHAPTER 13

Prevent Discharge Disasters

N EARLY ONE IN EVERY FIVE Medicare patients discharged from the hospital today is readmitted within 30 days, costing the U.S. healthcare system $26 billion annually. (1,2) The reasons for the high rate of readmissions are varied: lack of information provided to the patient during the discharge process, limited access to follow-up care, poor coordination between the hospital and outside providers, and adverse medication events.

To address these frequent and costly readmissions, hospitals and healthcare systems have developed coordinated action plans. One of the most frequently identified areas of concern lies with developing a detailed discharge process. Some hospitals have used nurse advocates to arrange timely follow-up appointments. Pharmacists have been enlisted to provide medication reconciliation to ensure consistency between what is prescribed in the hospital and what the patient will be taking at home. Post-discharge processes have been improved to include pharmacist callbacks to monitor and ensure appropriate medication use and compliance. There are even programs to maximize the use of health information technology to monitor patients in their homes via telehealth and transmit clinical data to their providers.

In addition to improving the discharge process, efforts to target high-risk patient populations *upon admission* is also underway. These efforts include improved admission processes to identify and stratify high-risk patients for a future risk of readmission and provide a multi-disciplinary team approach to optimize acute care while the patient is in the hospital. In addition, patients prescribed high-risk medications are identified when the medications are initiated to create a discharge regimen that will ensure adherence, decrease pill-burden, and even assist with the financial impact of post-discharge drugs. (5)

While government agencies focus on the high rates of hospital readmission and the associated exorbitant healthcare costs, providers are more appropriately troubled about the large gap in the transition of medical care from the hospital to the home leading to serious patient harm and often, deadly outcomes. Healthcare providers, including physicians, pharmacists, nurses, and others, constantly work to eliminate this gap to ensure the safety of their patients.

THE SUCCESSFUL DISCHARGE STRATEGY

A successful hospital discharge plan requires the coordinated efforts of the physician, nurse, pharmacist, patient, caregivers, and an assortment of various community services. A lack of coordination of this complex and integrated process is often the cause of serious post-discharge events and preventable, risky readmissions.

The typical discharge process can be fraught with pitfalls that patients need to anticipate and avoid. (1) These pitfalls can happen when patients are being transferred from the hospital to another facility (long-term care, rehabilitation, or hospice) or going home. These pitfalls can include: (1)

1. Not having a plan of care that details specific medical care needs, including equipment required, changes in diet, medication changes, as well as an assessment of the caregiver's ability to provide the necessary care.
2. Lack of primary care provider follow up within one week to assess overall recovery, adjust medications, respond to side effects and adverse reactions, and answer questions about the patient's care needs.
3. Lack of medication reconciliation between the pre-hospital and post discharge medications leading to therapeutic duplications and other adverse drug events.
4. Lack of communication with the caregiver, leading to confusion especially with changing wound dressings, administering injectable medications, or transferring the patient from wheelchair to bed.
5. Lack of support from family and other outside sources may lead to improper management of pain, anticoagulant therapy, physical therapy, etc. Caregivers often need to seek support from the physician or their staff to find solutions to specific issues that arise following discharge.

In isolation, any one of these serious situations could lead to confusion and errors, but if combined, they often leave patients and their caregivers frightened, confused, and back in the emergency department. A complete, coordinated, and standardized approach to the discharge process that bridges the gap from the patient's day of discharge to their first visit with their primary care provider is necessary to prevent this needless confusion and concern.

PROJECT RED

According to a study published in the *Annals of Internal Medicine*, patients who had a thorough understanding of their discharge instructions, including proper medication management and when to make follow-up appointments, had a 30% less chance of being readmitted or visit the emergency department within 30 days of discharge. (2)

To address the specific challenges of the discharge process, The Re-Engineered Hospital Discharge program (Project RED) was developed for the Agency for Healthcare Research and Quality (AHRQ) by Brian Jack, M.D., Associate Professor of Family Medicine at Boston University and Timothy Bickmore, Ph.D., Assistant Professor in the College of Computer and Information Science at Northeastern University.

Project RED has been shown to decrease hospital readmissions by using a nurse discharge advocate who follows a set of mutually reinforcing components leading to a safe and successful hospital discharge. (3) These components include:

1. Educating patients about their diagnosis throughout the hospital stay;
2. Making appointments for follow up and post-discharge testing, with input from patient about date and time;
3. Discussing with patient about any tests not completed in the hospital;
4. Organizing post-discharge services;
5. Confirming the medication plan;
6. Reconciling the discharge plan with national guidelines and critical pathways;
7. Reviewing with patient the appropriate steps to take in the event a problem arises;
8. Expediting transmission of the discharge summary to clinicians accepting care of the patient;
9. Assessing the patient's understanding of the plan;
10. Providing the patient with a written discharge plan; and
11. Calling the patient 2–3 days after discharge to reinforce the discharge plan and help with problem-solving.

In addition to the nurse discharge advocate, Project RED includes a patient-specific After Hospital Care Plan (AHCP) that clearly provides the information patients need to prepare them for the days between discharge and the first visit with their primary care doctor and a medication review phone call from a clinical pharmacist several days after discharge.

Project RED has been shown to decrease hospital readmissions by 30% within 30 days of discharge. This equates to reducing one readmission or emergency department visit for every 7.3 patients receiving the intervention. Further, the difference between study groups in total cost was $149,995, or an average of $412 per person who received the intervention. This represents a 33.9% lower observed cost for the intervention group. With more that 38 million hospital discharges in the United States each year, this intervention can drastically reduce cost and greatly improve the overall quality of patient care. (3)

In addition to providing a successful discharge plan, patients and their caregivers should be made aware of the pitfalls they may encounter once they get home.

Actively involving the patient and caregiver in discharge discussions will help ensure that medications are taken as prescribed, dressings are changed correctly, and any problems will be addressed appropriately if and when they arise.

SIMPLE PATIENT DISCHARGE INSTRUCTIONS

- Patients should not leave the hospital without an updated, written list of medications from the physician, nurse, or pharmacist. This list should include all of the medications the patients will be taking when they get home.
- Patients should know which of their old medications they will continue to take when they get home and which ones they should dispose of.
- Pharmacists should be available to provide discharge counseling on all medications the patient will be taking at home. Patients need to be sure that they understand these instructions and should ask questions to get clarification if they do not. Using the teach-back method will help providers ensure patients understand the information provided.
- Upon review of the medication list with the physician, nurse, or pharmacist, patients should be sure they understand what the medications are for, how to take them, and any possible side effects. If patients are not able to do this, have their caregiver review the list of medications with the healthcare provider on their behalf.
- If the patient is not able to comprehend this information, ask the caregiver or advocate to be there when the patient is discharged. They can help by asking questions that may not occur to the patient. The caregiver should bring a pad of paper and a pen to write down all of the important discharge information.
- Patients should know if they should avoid combining any prescription medications with any over-the-counter drugs, vitamins, dietary supplements, or herbal products. Many of these products can cause serious reactions with prescription medications, so patients should ask the pharmacist before taking any non-prescription agents.
- Many drugs, including sedatives and narcotics, interact with alcohol and medical marijuana and should not be taken together. Patients need to know if there are any foods or drinks, including alcoholic beverages, that should be avoided while taking these medications.
- Patients need to know what side effects to expect. They should also know what to do if they experience a side effect, allergic reaction, or other adverse event (including missing doses or doubling up).
- Patients should get their prescriptions filled as soon as possible after leaving the hospital. Serious errors will be prevented by starting new medications according to the schedule provided during the discharge process.

COORDINATED DISCHARGE CARE

- Begin with the end in mind. Upon admission, identify a healthcare professional to manage post-discharge care. (4)
- Screen and stratify patients upon admission for readmission risk, including disease states and high-risk medications. (5)
- Encourage multi-disciplinary daily rounds where all relevant clinicians address both acute care and a discharge regimen. (5)
- Provide clear, detailed discharge plans with considerations for health literacy and primary language spoken. (5)
- Engage patients and families in discharge planning and instructions. (5)
- Provide discharge instructions that meet the patient and caregiver's needs. (5)
- Identify follow up providers who can meet unique needs of the patient. (5)
- Arrange to have nurse discharge advocates coordinate timely follow-up appointments to primary care providers with the patient's convenience in mind. (2)
- Arrange to have nurse discharge advocates arrange timely access to community care services. (4)
- Ensure that medication reconciliation is completed and that all pre-admission medications are compared to post-discharge medications.
- Provide follow-up phone calls from a clinical pharmacist within several days post-discharge to ensure compliance with therapy and to address any medication issues. (2)
- Provide discharge services on weekends, nights, and holidays. (4)
- Identify patients at high risk for readmission and connect them to additional discharge support. (4)

BOTTOM LINE

Leveraging multidisciplinary care and pharmacy services will help patients avoid post-discharge adverse events and dangerous and costly hospital readmissions. Before patients leave the hospital, be certain that they have the information they need, including written instructions that they can refer to after they get home. Have patients speak with the nurse, doctor, or pharmacist about their medications and follow-up care. Be sure patients understand these instructions and follow them closely to prevent a rapid return to their hospital bed.

References

1. Irving C. Five common pitfalls of the hospital discharge process. Family Caregiver Alliance. http://blog.caregiver.org/?p=2040.
2. Jack BW, Chetty VK, Anthony D, et al. A reengineered hospital discharge program to decrease rehospitalization: a randomized trial. *Ann Intern Med.* 2009 Feb 3;150(3):178–187.

3. Jack B, Bickmore T. The re-engineered hospital discharge program to decrease rehospitalization. *CareManagement.* 2010 Dec/2011 Jan: 12–14.

4. National Priorities Partnership/NEHI. Preventing Hospital Readmission: A $25 Billion Opportunity. Cambridge, MA: NEHI, 2010.

5. The Joint Commission. *Advancing Effective Communication, Cultural Competence, and Patient and Family Centered Care: A Roadmap for Hospitals.* Oakbrook Terrace, IL: The Joint Commission, 2010.

CHAPTER 14

A Smooth Transition

A STUDY BY THE AGENCY FOR Healthcare Research and Quality (AHRQ) found that more than one-third of the patients who leave the hospital don't receive the follow-up care they need, such as follow-up lab tests or referrals to specialists. (1)

This is especially true for patients at high-risk of readmission, including those with congestive heart failure (CHF), chronic obstructive pulmonary disease (COPD), pneumonia, acute myocardial infarction (AMI), coronary artery bypass graft (CABG), and those on high-risk medications such as warfarin or insulin. With the increased number of patients with multiple comorbidities, limited health literacy, and age-related disorders, and fewer resources to care for them, it is easy to see why one in every five discharged patients is readmitted to the hospital within 30 days.

Hospitals are currently redesigning the discharge process to include age- and literacy-based education materials, nurse discharge advocates and social workers to coordinate community services, pharmacists to perform medication reconciliation, discharge counseling, and specialized training of insulin and other injections. It has been shown that patients who are discharged from the hospital with a clear understanding of their after-hospital care instructions, including how to take their medicines and when to make follow-up appointments, are 30% less likely to be readmitted or visit the emergency department than patients who lack this information. (1)

Despite these important initiatives, what actually happens when patients *get* home may be a totally different story. In reality, many patients are clearly unable to grasp the complexity and quantity of information that they are presented at discharge or perform the tasks they are expected to do. Patients with very complex treatment regimens may be under the care of an elderly spouse, a child living a long distance away, or a well-meaning family friend. Patients may rely on these caregivers to administer injections or inhaled medications, fill pill boxes, change wound dressings, insert catheters, or maintain oxygen supply, in addition to routine feeding, bathing and toileting, and transporting to follow-up appointments. Despite a well-coordinated discharge effort, patients find themselves acutely ill and back in the emergency department within days of going home.

PROVIDING A CLEAR ACTION PLAN

The AHRQ has developed *Taking Care of Myself: A Guide for When I Leave the Hospital* (2) that providers can give patients to help them manage their care after they get home. The guide includes specific information about why the patient was initially admitted and what to do/whom to call if a problem arises. It also includes medication lists for routine prescription drugs as well as "prn" or as-needed meds. There are several spaces for writing in questions prior to the follow-up office visits and a space for notes and comments. Download the complete form at: www.ahrq.gov

In addition:

- Provide a clear, step-by-step action plan for patients to follow after they get home. Patients may require an extremely detailed daily schedule with specific actions to take at various times of the day.
- Include the provider's name (or designated contact person) and phone number, including after-hours, cell phone, and pager numbers so the provider can be contacted if a problem or question arises.
- Include the names and phone numbers of any other healthcare professionals caring for the patient, such as the pharmacist, nurse practitioner, diabetes educator, anticoagulation clinic personnel, etc., whom the patient may contact with specific questions related to that particular illness or drug. This will prevent unnecessary calls to providers.
- Clearly define for the patient what an "adverse medication reaction" would be and what to do if this occurs. This may include a pharmacologic effect of the drug such as bleeding or bruising, but it may also include allergic reactions such as rash, edema, or shortness of breath.
- When possible, have prescriptions filled by the hospital pharmacy and delivered by pharmacy staff to the patient's bedside before discharge. Pharmacists should provide thorough discharge counseling to answer any questions the patient may have before going home. If this is not possible, make sure all prescriptions are called to a local pharmacy before discharge so the pharmacist can clarify any issues and the patient can pick them up as soon as possible.
- For patients starting warfarin therapy, make sure the follow-up appointment is scheduled for two or three days post-discharge. Patients sometimes "fall through the cracks" (with a subsequent readmission due to a perilously high INR) when they do not know to make a follow-up appointment with the anticoagulation clinic providers.
- Provide patients with the name and phone number of the contact at the anticoagulation clinic. Ask patients to contact the anticoagulation clinic if they do not hear from them in two days and schedule an appointment for follow up.

- For patients newly started on insulin therapy, be sure that the diabetes educator provides counseling prior to discharge and that the patients have the educator's contact information for any questions at home.
- Caregivers for patients who are sent home with a prescription for an injectable low-molecular weight heparin agent or other injectable drug need to be instructed on proper administration technique before leaving the hospital. It also may be beneficial to provide home-health nursing for the first few days to be sure the patient and/or caregiver is comfortable injecting this drug.
- Patients with COPD may be using several inhalers at once. Before discharge from the hospital, ask the pharmacist to review the name of each inhaler, what it is used for, and how it should be administered. Use this time as a "teachable moment" and ask the patient to demonstrate inhaler technique back to you.

BOTTOM LINE

Optimizing the transition of care from the hospital to home by providing clear after-care instructions is only part of the battle. Ensuring that the patient and their caregivers carry out these instructions is essential to reducing emergency room visits and hospital readmissions.

References

1. Agency for Healthcare Research and Quality. Preventing avoidable readmissions: improving the hospital discharge process. Agency for Healthcare Research and Quality. http://www.ahrq.gov/professionals/quality-patient-safety/patient-safety-resources/resources/impptdis/index.html. Accessed April 22, 2013.
2. Agency for Healthcare Research and Quality. Taking care of myself: a guide for when I leave the hospital. Agency for Healthcare Research and Quality. http://www.ahrq.gov/patients-consumers/diagnosis-treatment/hospitals-clinics/goinghome/index.html. Accessed April 22, 2013.

CHAPTER 15

Patient-Centered Medical Homes

THE PATIENT-CENTERED MEDICAL HOME MODEL (PCMH) is a new initiative aimed at transforming the way primary care is delivered in the United States. In 2007, four major physician organizations, including the American Academy of Family Physicians, the American Academy of Pediatrics, the American College of Physicians, and the American Osteopathic Association, endorsed the principles of PCMH.

According to the Agency for Healthcare Research and Quality (AHRQ), a medical home is a coordinated, patient-centered, multi-disciplinary approach to delivering the core functions of primary care. (1) These core functions include:

1. **Comprehensive Care:** Includes acute care, prevention, wellness, and chronic care. A team of providers, including physicians, nurses, pharmacists, nutritionists, social workers, educators, and care coordinator, provide this care.

2. **Patient-Centered:** Medical care that is relationship-based and focuses on the whole person. The patient-centered philosophy includes a physician who understands and respects the patient's unique needs, culture, values, and preferences. It also requires the patient and caregivers to learn to manage and organize their own care at a level they can manage and ensures that they are full partners in establishing care plans.

3. **Coordinated Care:** Across specialties, hospitals, home health, and community services. This is essential during critical transition times such as after hospital discharge.

4. **Accessible Services:** Includes shorter wait times for urgent needs, enhanced in-person hours, around-the-clock telephone or electronic access to a member of the care team, and alternative communication such as email and telephone consultation.

5. **Quality and Safety:** Using evidence-based medicine and clinical decision-support tools to guide shared decision making with patient and families. This model encourages the participation in performance improvement activities regarding patient experiences and satisfaction and population health management.

PCMH NATIONAL DEMONSTRATION PROJECT

In June 2006, the American Academy of Family Physicians initiated a national demonstration project (NDP) to test the PCMH in a sample of 36 family practices. (2) Early lessons from the NDP raised some serious concerns about the widespread implementation of medical homes, including underestimating the amount of time necessary for required changes, overestimating the readiness of technological advances, and serious undercapitalization.

The initial lessons learned from the NDP found that while most current medical practices are designed to enhance physician workflow, the PCMH is designed to enhance patient access and experience. This shift required an epic whole-practice transformation, not a quick quality-improvement initiative. It required new scheduling and access arrangements, new coordination arrangements with other parts of the healthcare system, group visits, new ways of bringing evidence to the point of care, quality improvement activities, institution of more point-of-care services, development of team-based care, changes in practice management, new strategies for patient engagement, and multiple new uses of information systems and technology. (2)

In addition to implementing new technology and office management strategies, physicians needed to change the way they approached patient care. This shift involved the move from physician-centered care to the team approach in which patient care is shared among trained staff. (3) This required not only trained, competent, and reliable clinical partners, but also facilitative leadership skills on behalf of the primary care physician instead of the traditional authoritarian focus. The PCMH expanded clinical care from the single-patient to population-based approach, especially for chronic diseases and preventative care. (4,5) Lastly, the PCMH required that physicians work in relationship-centered partnerships rather than just adhering to clinical guidelines. (6,7,8)

The Veterans Health Administration (VHA) is in the process of transforming the current method of delivering primary care from the traditional model to the patient-centered medical home model. The VHA is the largest integrated healthcare system in the United States, providing and paying for comprehensive care to over 5 million veterans each year. The VHA is a leader in innovation of electronic medical records, quality improvement, and cost control. (9) In 2010, the VHA initiated one of the largest PCMH programs to date. This included the transformation of over 850 hospital-based medical centers and community-based outpatient clinics to PCMH by the end of 2014.

The focus of the early PCMH implementation was on training pilot teams, funding additional staff, leveraging existing space and technology resources, and redesigning existing processes. In an evaluation of the first 18 months of implementation of strategies to improve access, including a focus on decreasing the demand for face-to-face care, increasing the supply of different types of primary care encounters, and improving clinic efficiencies, staff revealed three key issues that impacted their success. The VHA found that leadership engagement, staffing resources, and access to information had a significant impact on the overall readiness for PCMH implementation. (9)

PCMH requires a firm commitment from senior leadership down to the clerical staff. It also requires adequate resources and training and the acknowledgement that there may be a need for an "adaptive reserve" or time and resources as practices shift from current reactionary clinics to proactive prepared care teams. The ultimate goal of PCMH is to shift away from acute and chronic issues to prevention and changes to healthy behaviors, thus leading to improved outcomes and patient satisfaction.

THE PATIENT-CENTERED MEDICAL HOME TRANSFORMATION

- Engage leadership and stress managerial patience, "taking the long-term view to allow time for the often inevitable reduction in productivity" as pilot teams endeavor to test and implement new interventions. (10)
- Involve staff who have the technological expertise to access and make use of data to support change efforts.
- Assure adequate financial resources to cover new personnel, new technology, and ongoing operational dollars.
- Involve each practice in their individual model specifications. While practices may utilize outside resources for assistance, each practice should ultimately determine the time and amount of change for each step. (2)
- Provide physicians with facilitative leadership skill training if necessary. This can include working in teams, implementing change management, and partnering with patients. (2)
- Approach PCMH as a practice evolution, not a quick quality-improvement initiative. Transformation is a difficult and lengthy process and will need enhanced communication and adaptability to fully succeed. (2)
- Before beginning, research available technologies that best suit your practice.
- Continue to re-energize and motivate staff to prevent change fatigue and burnout.

BOTTOM LINE

The patient-centered medical home is the new model of primary care; however, it is imperative that practices view this as a transformation not a quick fix. Practices must ensure leadership engagement, adequate funding, and technological support before starting this process.

References

1. Agency for Healthcare Research and Quality. Patient centered medical home research center. Agency for Healthcare Research and Quality. *h*ttp://pcmh.ahrq.gov/portal/server.pt/community/pcmh_home/1483/PCMH_Defining%20t. Accessed January 6, 2013.

2. Nutting PA, Miller WL et. al., Initial Lessons From the First National Demonstration Project on Practice Transformation to a Patient-Centered Medical Home. Ann Fam Med 2009; 7: 254-260.

3. Grumbach K, Bodenheimer T. Can health care teams improve primary care practice? *JAMA.* 2004 Mar 10;291(10):1246–1251.

4. Bodenheimer T, Wagner EH, Grumbach K. Improving primary care for patients with chronic illness. *JAMA.* 2002 Oct 9;288(14):1775–1779.

5. Bodenheimer T, Wagner EH, Grumbach K. Improving primary care for patients with chronic illness: the chronic care model, Part 2. *JAMA.*2002 Oct 16; 288(15):1909–1914.

6. Brody H. Relationship-centered care: beyond the finishing school. *J Am Board Fam Pract.* 1995 Sep-Oct;8(5):416–418.

7. Marvel MK et. al., Soliciting the patient's agenda: have we improved? JAMA, 1999: 281 (3) 283-287.

8. Pew-Fetzer Task Force. *Health Professions Education and Relationship-centered Care.* San Francisco, CA: Pew Health Professions Commission, 1994.

9. True G, Butler AE, Lamparska BG, et al. Open access in the patient-centered medical home: lessons from the Veterans Health Administration. *J Gen Intern Med.* 2013 Apr;28(4):539–545. doi: 10.1007/s11606-012-2279-y.

10. Damschroder LJ, Aron DC, Keith RE, et al. Fostering implementation of health services research findings into practice: a consolidated framework for advancing implementation science. *Implement Sci.* 2009 Aug 7;4:50. doi: 10.1186/1748-5908-4-50.

CHAPTER 16

Can You Hear Me Now?

TELEHEALTH IS THE USE of telecommunications and information technology to provide access to health assessment, diagnosis, intervention, consultation, supervision, and other medical information across a distance. (1) Examples of telehealth include telephones, two-way video, videoconferencing, email, smart phones, wireless tools, transmission of still images, and ehealth such as patient portals, and remote patient monitoring devices.

Telemedicine is the exchange of medical information from one site to another using a variety of interactive telehealth applications. (2) Telemedicine seeks to improve patient care and patient access by permitting two-way, real-time interactive communication between the provider and patient at a remote site. Telemedicine is considered to be a cost-effective and convenient alternative to a traditional face-to-face examination.

Telemedicine provides a variety of services, including specialist referrals, patient consultations, remote patient monitoring or home telehealth, medical education, and consumer medical and health information. (2) These services are delivered using a number of different delivery mechanisms such as networked programs from hospitals to outlying clinics and health centers, point-to-point communication networks from hospitals and clinics contracting out to private providers at ambulatory care sites, primary or specialty care to the home, home to monitoring center, and web-based ehealth patient service sites. (2)

Telemedicine has been growing primarily in the areas that have a direct impact on the physician-patient partnership. These areas include home healthcare and disease management monitoring and remote doctor and specialist services. (3) Telemedicine has four essential benefits: 1) improved access, especially to patients in distant or rural locations; 2) cost effectiveness and improved efficiencies; 3) improved quality, particularly in mental health and ICU care; and 4) patient demand and improved satisfaction due to reduced travel time and access to medical services they might not have had otherwise. (4)

There are many different types of telemedicine specialty consultation services. These include allergy/immunology, anesthesia, cardiology, dermatology, emergency medicine, endocrinology, family practice, infectious disease, internal medicine,

71

mental health, neurology, and others. These consultations typically originate from healthcare systems, hospitals, or large medical group practices that employ a diverse collection of experts and highly trained specialists. (5) The specialists communicate with patients and/or providers at physically separate locations using technology to exchange medical information. The specialist examines the patient, orders labs and tests if necessary, and creates a consultation report for the referring physician. The specialist is generally reimbursed the same amount as if he or she had seen the patient in his or her own office. (5)

Reimbursement for telemedicine consultation can be equivalent to what is received for a face-to-face office visit. (6) Medicare allows billing for a limited set of live, interactive telemedicine services when the patient resides in a rural area, but will not reimburse for asynchronous or store-and-forward consultations. Store-and-forward consultations are those where there is a transfer of data from one site to another through the use of a camera that records (stores) an image that is sent (forwarded) via telecommunication to another site for consultation.

Medicare beneficiaries are eligible for telehealth services if they are presented from an "originating site" located in a rural health professional shortage area or in a county outside of a metropolitan statistical area. (7) Originating sites authorized by law are: offices of physicians or practitioners, hospitals, critical access hospitals (CAH), rural health clinics (RHC), federally qualified health centers (FQHC), hospital-based or CAH-based renal dialysis centers (including satellites), skilled nursing facilities (SNF), and community mental health centers (CMHC).

Practitioners at the distant site who may furnish and receive payment for covered telehealth services are: physicians, nurse practitioners, physician assistants, nurse midwives, clinical nurse specialists, clinical psychologists, clinical social workers, and registered dieticians or nutritional professionals. (7)

TELEMEDICINE ISSUES

There are telemedicine issues that are specific to certain types of facilities, those surveyed by different types of accrediting agencies (i.e., Joint Commission), and those dependent on certain payors such as Medicare or Medicaid.

Issues Specific to Provider Clinics

A rural physician clinic is an eligible originating site for CMS purposes. (8) Medicare patients seen by a specialist via telemedicine at a rural clinic are eligible for reimbursement. These clinics are not currently subject to Joint Commission standards, but CMS standards do apply. (8)

Issues Specific to Nursing Homes

Rural nursing homes are eligible originating sites for reimbursable telemedicine consultations. (8) This will help improve access to specialty care for frail and ill nursing home patients; however, nursing homes will now need to invest critical resources in telecommunications technology.

Issues Specific to Critical Access Hospitals

Telemedicine issues for critical access hospitals (CAH) are related to their remote, rural location and how they receive payment for Medicare-eligible patients. (8) Local costs of telemedicine may be incorporated into the cost basis used for determining Medicare payments and potential financial incentives are available through Medicare to provide certain consultation services. (8) CMS also has special policies related to physician reimbursement when the provider of the specialty service is located in a CAH. (9)

Issues Specific to Joint Commission-Accredited Hospitals

Joint Commission-accredited hospitals and other institutions are subject to medical staff standards regarding provider credentialing. A Joint Commission-accredited hospital maintains that the telemedicine provider must be credentialed and privileged at the organization where the patient is treated, and that the medical staff recommends the telemedicine services that are provided.

Exceptions to this rule include "consultations." Consultations, as defined for the purpose of credentialing and privileging requirements, are services provided by practitioners for the sole purpose of offering an expert opinion to and/or advising the treating practitioner, but not directing the patient's care. There are no specific Joint Commission credentialing and privileging requirements for specialists for these services. (8)

Exceptions for "interpretive services" also exist. Interpretive services are those services in which a licensed independent practitioner provides official readings of images, tracings, or specimens through a telemedicine link. (8) These include radiologists and pathologists and may include real-time services; or, the information can be transmitted using the store-and-forward technology.

THE EXPANDING ROLE OF TELEMEDICINE

- Before starting a telemedicine service, develop or adopt a protocol that clearly specifies how the service is to be conducted and evaluated. This protocol should include baseline measurements of performance criteria against which the service will be evaluated.

- Monitor telemedicine consultations and services periodically to ensure quality and consistency. A systematic plan should be used to monitor processes and strategies to ensure ongoing quality of care.
- Begin with outcomes in mind. Set straightforward goals at the outcome of the telemedicine service such as increased access, cost reduction, improved patient outcomes, and patient satisfaction, and have a process to ensure adequate measurement and tracking. (10)

BOTTOM LINE

Telemedicine may prove to be a cost-effective and convenient alternative to the traditional face-to-face way of providing medical care, for both the patient and provider. However, issues related to technology, training, reimbursement, and quality standards may need to be resolved before widespread use is attained.

References

1. Medicaid.gov. Telemedicine. *AMED News, Nov 13, 2012.* http://www.medicaid.gov. Accessed January 11, 2013.
2. American Telemedicine Association. Telemedicine defined. American Telemedicine Association. http://www.americantelemed.org/i4a/pages/index.cfm?pageid=3333. Accessed January 11, 2013.
3. Dolan, PL. Where growth is coming in telemedicine. American Medical Association. http://www.ama-assn.org/amednews/2012/11/12/bisc1113.htm. Accessed January 11, 2013.
4. American Telemedicine Association. About telemedicine. American Telemedicine Association. http://www.americantelemed.org/i4a/pages/index?pageID=3308. Accessed January 11, 2013.
5. Telehealth Resource Centers. Types of telemedicine specialty consultation services. Telehealth Resource Centers. http:///www.telehealthresourcecenter.org/toolbox-module/types-telemedicine-specialty-consultation-services. Accessed January 11, 2013.
6. Telehealth Resource Centers. Billing. Telehealth Resource Centers. http:///www.telehealth resourcecenter.org/toolbox-module/billing. Accessed January 11, 2013.
7. Department of Health and Human Services. Telehealth services on the Centers for Medicare and Medicaid Services (CMS) website. Department of Health and Human Services. http:///www.cms.gov/Medicare/Medicare-General-Information/Telehealth. Accessed January 11, 2013.
8. Telehealth Resource Centers. Issues specific to certain types of health organizations. Telehealth Resource Centers. http://www.telehealthresourcecenter.org/toolbox-module/issues-specific-certain-types-health-organizations. Accessed January 11, 2013.
9. Illinois Department of Public Health, Center for Rural Health. Critical access hospital telehealth network. National Rural Health Resource Center. http://www.ruralcenter.org/sites/default/files/telemed_network_description.pdf. Accessed January 13, 2013.
10. Telehealth Resource Centers. Evaluation. Telehealth Resource Centers. http://www.telehealth resourcecenter.ore/toolbox-module/evaluation. Accessed January 13, 2013.

CHAPTER 17

All Hands on Deck!

I T IS ESTIMATED THAT NEARLY 45% of the population of the United States is living with *at least one* chronic disease. (1) In 2003, more than 162 million cases of cancer, diabetes, heart disease, hypertension, stroke, mental disorders, and pulmonary conditions were reported. (2) In its study, *An Unhealthy America: The Economic Burden of Chronic Disease*, the Milken Institute reported the financial impact that chronic disease had on the U. S. economy. They found that treatment expenditures for these chronic illnesses accounted for over $277 billion annually (non-institutionalized) and over $1,046 billion in lost productivity, for a total cost over $1,323 billion annually. (2) As the population ages, these numbers are expected to rise with subsequent hospital admissions and readmissions. By 2030, it is estimated that there will be over 171 million chronically ill people living in the United States. (3)

From a therapeutic as well as financial standpoint, the treatment and prevention of chronic illnesses should be among the top priorities of U.S. healthcare providers. However, expecting practitioners to continually do more and more to effectively diagnose, treat, and monitor patients with complex chronic illnesses is particularly unreasonable. For this reason, the manner in which chronic illness is addressed in this country may need to be fundamentally changed.

THE CHRONIC CARE MODEL

The chronic care model (CCM) developed by Dr. Ed Wagner, M.D., (4) is a widely adopted approach to improving ambulatory care that targets chronic disease management on six distinct levels. The CCM is an integrated framework for practice redesign and includes:
1. Community resources;
2. Health-system organization;
3. Patient self-management and empowerment;
4. Delivery system design;
5. Clinical decision support; and
6. Clinical information systems.

The basis of the CCM is to increase providers' expertise and skill, educate and support patients, make care delivery more team-based and planned, and make better use of registry-based information systems. The CCM has been widely used in ambulatory care practices and provides the foundation for many patient-centered medical home models.

Several studies have shown that patients in practices where chronic disease management had been implemented received improved care. Patients with congestive heart failure (CHF) whose providers participated in the CHF disease management collaborative demonstrated a higher use of recommended medication therapies, lower use of the emergency department, 35% fewer days in the hospital, and an overall increased knowledge of their disease. (5)

For patients with asthma, those in practices where the chronic care model had been implemented were more likely to monitor peak flows, have a written action plan, and have an improved quality of life. (6) Lastly, diabetic patients who received care in a practice with the chronic care model experienced a reduced risk of cardiovascular disease; for every 48 patients who received care utilizing a chronic care model, the risk declined by one cardiovascular disease event. (7)

However, several more studies did not find such positive results. In a review of medical records of a random sample of diabetic patients in the years before, during and after the health collaborative, Chin and colleagues found that there was a significant improvement in the processes of care but not in the intermediate outcomes. (8) In a similar sample of patients with asthma and diabetes, Landon and colleagues found significantly greater improvements in process measures such as the use of anti-inflammatory medications for asthma and foot screening for diabetics in the year after the completion of the collaborative than did patients not in the collaborative. However, they found no difference in the intermediate outcomes such as hemoglobin A1c or blood pressure levels. (9)

In an effort to clarify these findings, in a second study, Chin and colleagues expanded the average time a patient was followed after the intervention from one year to three years. (10) They found again, that only process improvements were detected immediately after the collaborative. However, they also found that after two years, a significant improvement had been made in the intermediate outcomes such as HbA1c and low-density lipoprotein levels. These results supported the finding that the CCM was effective for improving care processes but also found that improvements in clinical outcomes requires additional time to emerge.

COORDINATED CARE

Effective chronic disease management may require the expertise of a coordinated multidisciplinary team. This team may include the primary care doctor and the nurse, and may also include specialists, pharmacists, diabetic educators, nutritionists, nurse case managers, home health nurses, and community health care workers, just to name a few. Clinical pharmacists and specialized nurses are routinely involved in the care and medication management of patients on anticoagulants, lipid therapy, treatment of heart disease, diabetic therapy, hepatitis C, pain management, mental health issues, chronic obstructive pulmonary disease, congestive heart failure, cancer, hypertension, stroke, and others. Providers need to avail themselves of these resources and involve as many experts as possible in the care, treatment and monitoring of patients with chronic disease.

In addition to the healthcare team, patients themselves may be a major contributor in their own care. In chronic illness, patients need to be aware that the goal is not a cure, but the establishment of a "new normal" that incorporates the illness into the patient's everyday routine. Patients need to know and understand the limitations of the disease, including self-management of medications, pain control, behavior modifications, and coping with differing situations and events. (11)

Patients may also benefit from group visits with their primary care provider where they are able to share concerns and problems they are having with their disease. Lastly, the use of telehealth or other remote therapeutic management may be beneficial to maintain communication with patients, provide continuous monitoring, and prevent any potential errors. (11)

CHRONIC DISEASE MANAGEMENT

- Take an "all hands on deck" approach to the management of chronic disease by using teams of doctors, pharmacists, nurses, and community services.
- Ensure that critical elements of care are performed competently, including regulation of medications, self-management support, and thorough follow up.
- Include patients as partners in chronic disease management. Patients themselves may provide necessary contribution to their own healthcare.
- Promote prevention and early intervention as a means to stopping chronic disease.
- Work with government agencies, insurers, and employers to incentivize patients for choosing healthy lifestyle choices. These programs may include smoking cessation, weight loss, exercise and fitness, and prevention of drug and alcohol abuse.

BOTTOM LINE

The personal and financial impact of chronic illness in the United States is almost immeasurable. Prevention is the ultimate goal; however, treatment strategies using teams of healthcare providers, as well as the patients themselves, may offer the most effective approach.

References

1. Wu, S, Green A. *Projection of chronic illness prevalence and cost inflation.* Santa Monica, CA: RAND, October 2000.

2. DeVol R, Bedroussian A, et al. *An unhealthy America: the economic burden of chronic disease. Charting a new course to save lives and increase productivity and economic growth.* Santa Monica, CA: Milken Institute, October 2007. http://www.milkeninstitute.org/pdf/ES_ResearchFindings.pdf

3. Improving Chronic Illness Care. http://www.improvingchroniccare.org.

4. Coleman K, Austin B, Brach C, Wagner E. Evidence on the chronic care model in the new millennium. *Health Aff* (Millwood). 2009 Jan-Feb;28(1):75-85. doi: 10.1377/hlthaff.28.1.75.

5. Asch SM, Baker, DW, Keesey JW, et al. Does the collaborative model improve care for chronic heart failure? *Med Care.* 2005 Jul;43(7):667-675.

6. Mangione-Smith R, Schonlau M, Chan KS, et al. Measuring the effectiveness of a collaborative for quality improvement in pediatric asthma care: does implementing the chronic care model improve processes and outcomes of care? *Ambul Pediatr.* 2005 Mar-Apr;5(2):75-82.

7. Vargas RB, Mangione CM, Asch S, et al. Can a chronic care model collaborative reduce heart disease risk in patients with diabetes? *J Gen Intern Med.* 2007 Feb;22(2):215-222.

8. Chin MH, Cook S, Drum ML, et al. Improving diabetes care in midwest community health centers with the health disparities collaborative. *Diabetes Care.* 2004 Jan;27(1):2-8.

9. Landon BE, Hicks LS, O'Malley AJ et al. Improving the management of chronic disease at community health centers. *N Engl J Med.* 2007 Mar 1;356(9):921-934.

10. Chin MH, Drum ML, Guillen M, et al. Improving and sustaining diabetes care in community health centers with the health disparities collaboratives. *Med Care.* 2007 Dec;45(12):1135-43.

11. Holman H, Lorig K, Patients as partners in managing chronic disease. *BMJ, 2000;320:526-7.*

CHAPTER 18

HAM It Up!
(High-Alert Medications)

STUDIES HAVE SHOWN THAT ADVERSE MEDICATION EVENTS are a major contributor to hospital readmissions. (1) Despite the fact that medications are considered one of the most common, safest, and effective interventions in healthcare, not all medications are safe for all patients.(2) The Institute for Safe Medication Practice has identified a list of medications considered "high-alert" medications (HAMs). (3) These medications are associated with more harm than other medications. They not only cause harm more frequently, the harm they produce is considerably more serious than other medications. High-alert medications also have the highest risk for causing injury if they are misused. The Institute for Healthcare Improvement found that focusing on four groups of medications has the greatest impact on reducing patient harm and subsequent hospital readmissions. (4) These four groups are considered to be high-alert medications: 1) anticoagulants, 2) narcotics, 3) sedatives, and 4) insulin.

ANTICOAGULANTS

Heparin, low-molecular weight heparin, and warfarin all play a vital role in anticoagulant and antithrombotic therapy, especially for atrial fibrillation, deep vein thrombosis, pulmonary embolism, and mechanical heart valve implant. Proper use of these agents is critical to ensure safety and successful therapeutic outcomes; however, complex dosing, inadequate monitoring and follow up, and poor patient compliance often lead to poor outcomes and patient harm.

Studies have shown that anticoagulants account for 4% of all actual adverse drug events and 10% of all potential adverse drug events in the inpatient and outpatient settings. Warfarin alone is commonly implicated due to complex dosing, numerous food and drug interactions, and lack of patient compliance. (5,6)

Safety Tips for Anticoagulation Therapy

- Use approved order sets and protocols for initiation and maintenance of anticoagulation therapy.
- Require that pharmacists double-check all VTE prophylaxis therapy.

- Use protocols to discontinue or restart warfarin perioperatively.
- Use flow sheets that follow patients throughout all transitions of care (patient-based, not unit-based).
- Authorize nurses to administer rescue drugs based on protocol.
- Assess the patient's baseline coagulation status.
- Use only oral unit-dose products, prefilled syringes, or premixed infusion bags when available.
- Use low-molecular weight heparin where clinically appropriate instead of unfractionated heparin.
- Use a written policy to address baseline and ongoing lab tests.
- Ensure effective systems and processes are in place to ensure the timely reporting and review as well as the necessary action to take in the event of critical lab results.
- Allow pharmacists to change anticoagulant doses based on lab values per protocol.
- Reduce the number of heparin concentrations in the hospital and use prepackaged heparin infusions when possible.
- Use programmable infusion pumps for IV heparin therapy.
- Use pump alerts for dose monitoring. Be sure the staff does not ignore these alerts.
- Monitor anticoagulant therapy closely and act to mitigate any medication administration delays or omissions.
- Include pharmacists on rounds to adjust and monitor anticoagulant therapy.
- Use pharmacists to assist with the identification of alternatives when therapeutic or dietary interactions and contraindications exist.
- Perform automatic nutrition consults on all warfarin patients to prevent drug-food interactions.
- Manage food and drug interactions on an inpatient and outpatient basis.
- Transition patients to anticoagulant clinics after discharge for adequate monitoring.
- Limit warfarin to one tablet strength (on an outpatient basis) and dose adjust based on increments of that tablet strength (i.e. "Take one tablet (5mg) on Monday, Wednesday, and Friday and take ½ tablet (2.5mg) all other days") instead of dispensing two different tablet strengths to be taken on different days.
- Provide ongoing education to all prescribers, staff, patients, and families regarding anticoagulant therapy.
- Evaluate anticoagulation safety practices on a routine basis and take action to improve practices in a timely manner.

OPIOIDS

In a study led by the Child Health Corporation of America (CHCA) a rate of 5.2 narcotic-related adverse events occurred for every 100 hospitalized patients. (7) Adverse events attributed to opioid use included overdose with subsequent respiratory depression and underdose with poor pain control. Patient-controlled analgesia (PCA) also posed a potential for respiratory depression due to drug interactions, continuous narcotic infusion, and inappropriate use of PCA by patients. (8)

Safety Tips for Opioid Therapy

- Use order sets to prescribe narcotics, including dosing limits.
- Use "smart pumps" with an up-to-date drug library and perform a nursing double check all opioid IV infusions.
- Limit the number of drug concentrations and the volume of each narcotic infusion where appropriate.
- Use electronic alerts to prevent over-sedation and respiratory arrest.
- Use the data from the alerts and overrides to assess standards and redesign processes.
- Make staff aware of the errors associated with patient-controlled analgesia (PCA) pumps.
- Avoid the use of multiple narcotics.
- Use pharmacists to perform drug-conversion dosing.
- Perform a fall risk assessment on patients taking narcotics.
- Where available, refer patients on long-term opioid use to pain management and opioid renewal clinics for evaluation and follow-up monitoring.

SEDATIVES

Due to the many sedatives on the market today, clinicians may not be aware of the onset and duration of action of these agents. Additionally, knowledge of the side effects; upper dose limits, especially when titrating to effect; drug interactions (Rx and OTC); interactions with alcohol; and concurrent use with other anxiolytics and hypnotics may lead to serious patient harm.

Facilities may lack effective processes to address emergency situations such as respiratory depression or arrest that may occur with the use of these medications. Multiple sedative use as well as sedative use in the elderly is of particular concern by the Institute of Safe Medication Practices.

Safety Tips for Sedative Therapy

- Use order sets to prescribe sedatives, including age-adjusted dosing limits.
- Use alerts to prevent over-sedation and respiratory arrest.
- Avoid the use of multiple sedatives.
- Use pharmacists to perform accurate dosing and provide recommendations for alternative therapies.

- Minimize or eliminate multiple drug strengths and formulations of sedatives/hypnotics where possible.
- Monitor for the use of multiple sedatives, hypnotics, anxiolytics, antidepressants, or narcotics prescribed for one patient.
- Use non-pharmacological methods of sedative management where appropriate.
- Perform a fall risk assessment on patients taking sedatives.
- Where available, refer patients on long-term sedative use to mental health providers for evaluation and follow-up monitoring.

INSULIN

Hypoglycemia continues to be a frequent adverse event related to insulin therapy in hospitals worldwide. Due to the pharmacology of insulin (long-acting vs. short-acting), complexity of dosing (basal/bolus vs. sliding scale), and a number of different insulin products, there is the potential for error and consequent patient harm. Studies have shown that despite the use of insulin-dosing protocols and guidelines in place in most hospitals today, adverse events continue to occur.

Safety Tips for Insulin Therapy

- Develop standard order sets for insulin therapy using evidence-based therapeutic regimens.
- Link order sets to recent lab values.
- Allow nurses to administer rescue medications based on protocol (i.e., hypoglycemia).
- Reduce sliding scale variations or eliminate the use of sliding scale insulin therapy altogether.
- Minimize interruptions during process of insulin administration.
- Recommend nurses double check all insulin orders at time of administration.
- Closely coordinate insulin administration and meal times as well as the amount of meal consumed.
- Monitor overlapping insulin and oral hypoglycemic agents prescribed for one patient.
- Allow patient management of insulin therapy when appropriate.

SAFETY TIPS FOR HIGH-ALERT MEDICATIONS

- As per the Joint Commission recommendations, create a list of high-alert medications in your hospital and implement strategies to reduce the risk of adverse events associated with these medications.
- Create an awareness of high-alert medications, including insulin, opioids, anticoagulants, sedatives, and any other medications specific to your facility

or practice. Make these medications the focus of departmental and facility newsletters and medical staff meetings and campaigns. (2)

- Review the ISMP Action Agenda on a quarterly basis and implement strategies that are appropriate for your facility. Issues that are included in the ISMP Action Agenda are problems that have surfaced at other hospitals across the country and may be applicable to yours.
- Analyze facility-specific adverse drug event reports for high-alert medications, including medication errors, near misses, adverse drug reactions, missing dose reports, and others. Perform root-cause analysis or failure mode-effect analysis to determine why these errors occur. (2)
- Develop standardized order sets to help providers prescribe certain high-alert drugs. (2)
- Select the high-alert medication with the highest priority and begin to implement safety strategies instead of tackling all high-alert medications simultaneously.
- Create facility-specific alerts for high-alert medications such as storing them in red bins and affixing "High Alert" labels to the bins.
- If the facility has barcoding capabilities, require the use of barcoding when administering high-alert medications.
- Require a double check by nursing staff before administration of high-alert medications.
- Do not allow the use of unacceptable abbreviations, especially with high-alert medications. This includes the use of "U" for units. Require providers to spell out the word "units," especially when prescribing insulin and heparin.

BOTTOM LINE

High-alert medications are associated with more patient harm than other medications. Standardization and customization of processes related to the prescribing, dispensing, and administration of individual high-alert medications will help prevent errors and needless patient harm.

References

1. Forster AJ, Clark HD, Menard A, et al. Adverse events among medical patients after discharge from hospital. *CMAJ*. 2004 Feb 3;170(3):345-349.
2. Health Research and Educational Trust. *Implementation guide to reducing harm from high-alert medications*. Chicago, IL: HRET, 2012.
3. Institute for Safe Medication Practices. *ISMP's list of high-alert medications*. Institute for Safe Medication Practices. http://www.ismp.org/tools/highalertmedications.pdf.
4. Institute for Healthcare Improvement. *How-to guide: Prevent harm from high-alert medications*. Cambridge, MA: Institute for Healthcare Improvement; 2012. www.ihi.org.

5. Bates DW, Cullen DJ, Laird N, Peterson LA , et al. Incidence of adverse drug events and potential adverse drug events. Implications for prevention. ADE Prevention Study Group. *JAMA*. 1995 Jul 5;274(1):29-34.

6. Kanjanarat P, Winterstein AG, Johns TE, et al. Nature of preventable adverse drug events in hospitals: a literature review. *Am J Health Syst Pharm*. 2003 Sep 1;60(17):1750-1759.

7. Child Health Corporation of America. CHCA Improvement Case Study.

8. Looi-Lyons LC, Chung FF, Chan VW, McQuestion M. Respiratory depression: an adverse outcome during patient controlled analgesia therapy. *J Clin Anesth*. 1996 Mar;8(2):151-156.

CHAPTER 19

The "Canary in the Coal Mine" Theory

ADHERENCE WITH MEDICATION REGIMENS is key to optimal patient outcomes. However, according to the National Association of Chain Drugstores, for every 100 prescriptions written, 50–70 actually go to the pharmacy, 48–66 come out of the pharmacy, 25–30 are taken properly, and 15–20 are refilled as prescribed. (1)

Nonadherence to treatment regimens accounts for 10%–25% of hospital admissions. (2) Research has found that nonadherence resulted in 5.4 times increased risk of hospitalization, rehospitalization, or premature death for patients with hypertension (3); 2.5 times increased risk of hospitalization for patients with diabetes; and more than 40% of nursing home admissions. (4)

Nonadherence results in an economic burden of $100 to $300 billion per year (5), with an increased annual cost of $2,000 per patient in physician visits. (6) The rate of medication nonadherence is expected to increase as the population ages and the burden of chronic illness increases.

Adherence to medication regimens depends on five interacting factors: (2)

1. **Social and Economic:** Low health literacy, lack of family or social support, homelessness, burdensome schedule, lack of access to healthcare facilities or pharmacies, lack of health insurance, and medication costs.
2. **Healthcare System:** Relationship between the patient and provider, provider communication skills, poor patient information materials, restrictive drug formularies, long wait times, and poor continuity of care.
3. **Condition-related:** Chronic illness, psychotic disorders, depression, severity of symptoms, or lack of symptoms.
4. **Therapy-related:** Complexity of medication regimen, treatment requiring mastery of certain techniques, duration of therapy, changes in therapy, side effects, treatment that interferes with lifestyle or requires behavioral change.
5. **Patient-related:** Physical—visual, hearing, or cognitive impairment; impaired dexterity; and swallowing problems. Psychological/behavioral—knowledge about illness, understanding why medication is needed, perceived benefit from

treatment, motivation, fear of dependence, frustration with providers, stress, anxiety, anger, alcohol or substance abuse.

MINIMALLY DISRUPTIVE MEDICINE

The concept of "minimally disruptive medicine" championed by Dr. Victor Montori, M.D., a diabetologist and researcher at the Mayo Clinic, is a new approach to treating medication nonadherence. Dr. Montori found that poor care coordination, increasingly complex medication regimens, and a shift toward patient self-management may increase the "work" of being chronically ill to a point that the patient cannot manage his or her own care. Dr. Montori states that reducing the "workload of chronic illness" especially for those with multiple illnesses, will lead to improved adherence and better outcomes.

Achieving minimally disruptive medicine requires that the practice of medicine redesigns effective treatment strategies for patients while minimizing the burden of treatment. This should lead to treatment programs that fit with patients' goals and lifestyles and that patients can make a "normal" part of their life. Dr. Montori likens the patient who stops showing up for appointments and taking medications when the burden of chronic illness becomes too much to handle to the "canary in the coal mine" who stops singing when conditions become toxic. He stresses that when patients stop showing up, its time to become concerned and take measures to ensure adherence to medications and other treatment regimens.

Dr. Montori states that so-called noncompliance is actually an alarm system for a healthcare system that is failing patients. The goal needs to be shifting and sharing responsibility for chronic disease *with* patients and families, not shifting the burden *onto* them.

WHAT YOUR PATIENTS NEED TO KNOW ABOUT TAKING MEDICATIONS SAFELY AND CORRECTLY

Organization is the key to medication management. However, this can be overwhelming, especially if your patients take many different medications at several different times of the day. Here are some pointers to help your patients take their medications safely and correctly:

Patient Safety Tips for Taking Medications Correctly

- Be sure to read the prescription label before you take the medication. You may think that you know how to take your medications, but check the label for any information that may be new, confusing, and unclear. If you are confused about how to take a medication, call the pharmacist first.

- Make sure you understand the directions on the label. Sometimes you might read the label, but still not know what to do. Confusing directions can lead to serious problems when the medication is taken incorrectly.
- Check the refill information before you run out of the medication. If you wait too long and there are no refills left, you may have to go for days without your medication while you wait for your doctor to authorize a refill. This may take several days. Your pharmacist can help you with refills, but you need to call in advance to allow plenty of time for the pharmacist to work with the doctor.
- Keep an updated list of your medications. This is the easiest way to stay organized. The medication list is where you will write in the names of all of your drugs, how you take them, and any side effects. It also has a place to write in your allergies. The medication list should include all prescriptions as well as over-the-counter, herbal, dietary supplements, natural products, vitamins, etc., that you take. Ask your pharmacist if you need help filling out your list.
- Create a medication-dosing schedule that lists all of the medications you take, how you take them, and when you take them. If you need help filling this out, ask your pharmacist for help.
- Make taking your pills part of your daily routine. For example, if you take your pills in the morning, make it a habit to take them after brushing your teeth or after eating your breakfast. Just be sure to match up the routines with the proper way to take the drugs. Some medications must not be taken together, must be taken with food, or must be taken at certain times. Your pharmacist can help you coordinate your medication schedule with your routines.
- If you take medication that is stored in the refrigerator, put a sticky note on the refrigerator door that says "Take Meds."
- If you take a medication with a meal, put the bottle on the table where you eat and be sure to take your pill when you finish eating. If you have small children around, be sure to put your pill bottles away in a locked cabinet when you're done.
- Set an alarm to signal when it is time to take your pills. Then take the medications when the alarm goes off—don't ignore it.
- Keep a daily pillbox that has separate compartments for each day of the week to help you stay organized and remember if you took your pills that day. Pillboxes come with varying numbers of compartments for different times of day (morning, noon, evening, and bedtime) and in different sizes to accommodate many different medication combinations, shapes, and sizes. Many pharmacies supply pillboxes at no charge. The major drawback to using pillboxes is that they are not childproof. Leaving the pillbox where a child could reach it can lead to accidental poisonings. Be sure to put it in a locked cabinet when children are in the house.
- Try a pill reminder gadget. These days, you can find many different types of gadgets to help you remember to take your pills (see below). These range from

simple alarms and voice reminders to automatic, lockable, pill dispensers. Some of the more advanced devices are expensive, but the cost may be offset by the peace of mind of knowing you are taking your medications correctly.

- If you are computer savvy or have a smart phone, you may want to use technology to help you take your meds on time. If you are on the computer for much of the day, you can set a computer-generated alert (like an electronic sticky note) to help you remember. You can also use your cell phone to set an alarm that will go off at a certain time each day or set cell phone calendars with recurring reminders to take your meds.
- Ask for help. Caregivers are a critical asset in helping you remember to take your meds. They can help you with your medication schedule and help you fill your pillbox.

Here is a partial list of great gadgets you can use to help remember to take your medications.

Automatic Pill Dispensers: Automatic electronic pill dispensers are convenient medication organizers that dispense the correct dose at the appropriate time, sounding an alarm to remind the person to take the medication. The caregiver loads and programs the dispenser. Some dispensers need to be refilled weekly, others every two weeks, and others on a monthly basis. Some dispensers alert a person to take their pills one to two times a day, while others will alert up to four times a day.

Many of these automatic pill dispensers are equipped with locks, so the person taking the pills cannot overdose. Some models record the time of day a pill was taken, display how often the pills were taken, and then provide this information to caregivers and doctors. These pillboxes even send an email, text message, or phone call to notify a remote caregiver if a medication dose was missed. These pillboxes are expensive and charge a monthly subscription fee.

Prices for the basic organizer with a timer start around $30. The more advanced models cost approximately $150.

Alarm Wristwatches: The alarm wristwatch is a nifty gadget that sets off an alarm when it is time to take your medications. You may program alarms to go off several times a day and set the alert for audio, vibrating, or even text message. Many of the watches also have room to store important medical information, such as medical history, allergies, blood type, and insurance information. The alarm wristwatches range in price from $30 to $100, depending on the features.

Prescription Bottle Caps with Alarms: You can set the alarm right on your prescription bottle with a special bottle cap that fits onto a standard prescription bottle. The alarm sounds when it is time to take your pills. Some caps include visual alerts like flashing lights or displays. Some caps even trigger an alert when you haven't taken your pills and will call you on your cell phone to remind you. Warning: Many of these prescription bottle caps are not childproof. Ask your pharmacist about these caps if you have children around the house.

"There's an app for that": If you are tech-savvy, you can find plenty of software applications to help remind you to take your meds. You can use these apps on your personal home computer, your smart phone or PDA, and even your office PC. Many of these programs include daily alarms that beep, send a text message to your computer screen, or even email you. The software includes neat features like medication lists, medication dosing schedules, a log of how often you took your medication (or missed it), and prescription refill reminders. Many of these software programs are free; some come with a monthly subscription fee. When you find one you like, check it out first to be sure there are no hidden costs and that your medical information will be secure.

BOTTOM LINE

Being a chronic patient is hard work, and providers must address the burden of illness when designing a successful treatment strategy. Adopt some of the simple strategies listed to help ease the burden of chronic illness.

References

1. National Association of Chain Drug Stores. *Pharmacies: improving health, reducing costs.* Arlington, VA: National Association of Chain Drug Stores, 2010.
2. American Society of Consultant Pharmacists. Adult medication. American Society of Consultant Pharmacists. http://www.adultmedication.com/downloads/Adult_Medication.pdf. Accessed April 22, 2013.
3. Gwadry-Sridhar FH, Manias E. Zhang Y, et al. A framework for planning and critiquing medication compliance and persistence research using prospective study designs. *Clin Ther.* 2009 Feb;31(2):421–435. doi: 10.1016/j.clinthera.2009.02.021.
4. Lau DT, Nau DP. Oral antihyperglycemic medication nonadherence and subsequent hospitalization among individuals with type 2 diabetes. *Diabetes Care.* 2004 Sep;27(9):2149–2153.
5. DeMatteo MR. Variations in patients' adherence to medical recommendations: a quantitative review of 50 years of research. *Med Care.* 2004 Mar;42(3):200–209.
6. American Pharmacists Association. *Medication compliance-adherence-persistence digest.* American Pharmacists Association. 2012: 1–12.

CHAPTER 20

"I Can't Even Afford a Free Meal"

A S A PHARMACIST, I have encountered many people who could not afford to pay for their medications. They have come to the pharmacy counter with a single dollar bill (sometime just the change in their pockets), trying to buy a day's worth of six to eight different medications just to get them by until the next paycheck. This is an extremely sad state of affairs but one that is all too common in pharmacies today. When people skip doses, cut pills in half (or thirds or fourths) to make them last, don't refill them, or just stop taking them, these people end up in emergency rooms much sicker than they were to start with. Pharmacists are in a key position and can suggest safe and practical ways to help patients save money on the prescription medications they so desperately need.

RXPERT ADVICE—ASK YOUR PHARMACIST FOR HELP

Joe's doctor was confused. According to Joe's medical chart, he was taking five different drugs. These were for arthritis, high cholesterol, diabetes, depression, and heartburn. However, when Joe was in the doctor's office that day for a checkup, his blood sugar was high, he was complaining of arthritis pain, and his acid reflux had gotten worse. The doctor asked Joe if he was taking all of his medications as prescribed. Joe said, "Oh yes, I take all of my medications every day, just like I'm supposed to."

Joe was thinking to himself, *Doc, the total bill for those five drugs is nearly $1,000 every month! There is no way that I can afford that. I am on a fixed income and my insurance doesn't cover drugs. Right now, I can't even afford a free meal. I haven't taken any medication for the past two months, and I'm afraid something bad is going to happen to me.*

The doctor thought that the medications Joe was taking were not working. He changed some of the drugs and increased the dose of the others. Joe went home with his new prescriptions. He did not even stop at the pharmacy. Why bother? He couldn't afford the new drugs any more than the old ones.

A few days later, Joe was admitted to the emergency department. He was nauseated and was having trouble breathing. The doctor in the ED treated Joe for high blood sugar and asked him what medication he was taking. Joe told the doctor that he had stopped taking all of his medications several months ago because he could not afford them. The doctor gave Joe a week's supply of medication and told him to see his doctor as soon as he could.

When Joe saw his primary care doctor, he admitted that he had stopped taking his medications. He simply could not afford them. The doctor reviewed Joe's medications and substituted low-cost generic medications or lower-cost therapeutic substitutions for the high-cost brand-name drugs he had originally prescribed. The pharmacist was able to fill them with the low-cost generic drugs that were on the $4 drug list. The total bill for an entire month's supply of medication was just $20! Joe was pleasantly surprised and very relieved. He could finally afford his medications and would take them as prescribed.

SIMPLE STEPS FOR CUTTING DRUG COSTS

- One of the simplest ways to safely lower drug costs is to use generic drugs. Pharmacists are aware of recent generic drug approvals or when a high-cost brand name drug will be available in generic form.
- Many pharmacies now offer generic medications for $4 for a month's supply. Have patients ask their pharmacist if the drug is on the $4 list.
- For chronic conditions like hyperlipidemia, hypertension, depression, and GERD, lower-cost alternative *brand-name* drugs are available in place of many high-cost brand-name medications. Typically, these drugs are older versions of newer, more expensive drugs. Some of these drugs may even be available as a generic, saving even more money! For example, several older statins like simvastatin and pravastatin have similar efficacy as the newer brand-name drugs and may work just as well for your patient.
- Many drugs that used to be available only by prescription are now available over the counter. These drugs include Prilosec, Prevacid, Zyrtec, Claritin, and others. Patients may be able to switch from the prescription product to one that is similar in an over-the-counter form. For example: A 30-day supply of prescription Nexium costs approximately $199.99 per month. Prilosec, available over-the-counter, costs approximately $22.89 for 42 tablets.*
- Tablet splitting or "half-tabs" may help your patients save money. Tablet splitting involves prescribing double the strength tablet required and then having the patient split the pill in half to get the correct dose. For example, a 20 mg tablet may cost the same as a 10 mg tablet, so your patient can save money

*Retail costs as of 11/2010.

by buying the 20 mg tablet and cutting it in half. However, if your patient is easily confused or does not have the manual dexterity to split tablets safely, this may not be appropriate. When prescribing half-tabs ask the pharmacist to instruct the patient on splitting the tablet and providing a "pill splitter" to get the correct dose.

- Most medications contain a single agent; however, combination drugs can help save your patients money and provide convenience. For example, hydrochlorothiazide and lisinopril come as a combination product rather than using two separate single agents. The combination drug may be more expensive if your patient pays out of pocket, but with a prescription drug co-pay, he or she will have to pay only one co-pay for the combination product. Ask the pharmacist if certain agents are available in combination form.

Drug Company Assistance Programs

- Drug company patient assistance programs (PAP) provide a limited number of brand-name medications to eligible patients at little or no cost. However, there are differences in the way these programs are designed, including the drugs that are covered, the application process, income criteria, co-pays, and the length of time covered. Ask patients to check with their pharmacists before signing up for a PAP or go to www.healthassistrx.com for more information about drug company programs.

- Several programs offer drug discount cards that can be used for medications that are 1) not covered by insurance, 2) have a high co-pay or deductible, 3) are applicable if the low medication cap has been reached, or 4) are applicable if they are in the Medicare Part D donut hole. The cards are not associated with an insurance plan and cannot be used in combination with Medicaid, Medicare, or other state or federal programs that pay for medications. However, patients can use the card if they are not using another program to pay for the drug. These cards are valid only at participating pharmacies and may be a good option for high-cost drugs not covered by an insurance plan. Patients can go to www.needymeds.org or www.Rxassist.org for more information regarding drug discount cards.

- Buying prescription drugs at a reputable online pharmacy may save a great deal of money. However, be sure that the pharmacy has the VIPPS seal of approval. This seal ensures that the pharmacy is a state-licensed pharmacy in good standing and located in the United States. These sites have undergone and successfully completed the National Association of Boards of Pharmacy (NABP) accreditation process.

- Herbal products, nutritional supplements, and natural remedies are not cheap. Some of these products sell for $30 or more a bottle. Unfortunately, most of these supplements have not been proven safe *or* effective. Additionally, many supplements and natural products can interact negatively with prescription drugs Instruct patients to play it safe and ask the pharmacist if a specific herbal product is safe for them to take. Otherwise, patients should save their money— these products could be doing them more harm than good.

Drug-Discount Card Programs

Many pharmaceutical companies offer discount cards that can save you money each year.

- Johnson and Johnson Partnership for Prescription Assistance—www.pparx. org. Phone: 888-4PPA-NOW
- Pfizer Pfriends Program—www.pfizerhelpfulanswers.com. Phone: 866-776-3700
- AstraZeneca Foundation Patient-Assistance Program—www.astrazeneca-us. com. Phone: 800-424-3727
- Lilly Answers—www.lilly.com. Phone: 800-545-6962
- Janssen Patient Assistance Program—www.janssen.com. Phone: 800-652-6227
- Medicare-Approved Drug Discount Cards—www.medicare.gov. Phone: 800-MEDICARE
- Together Rx Access—www.trxaccess.com. Phone: 800-444-4106

BOTTOM LINE

Using a generic drug, a lower-cost alternative, an over-the-counter agent, half-tabs, or combination products can help save your patients money. Additionally, drug company assistance programs may provide a valuable alternative. Have patients consult with their pharmacist to see if these options are right for them.

Minimize Medication Errors

"Drugs don't work in patients who don't take them."

C. EVERETT KOOP

CHAPTER 21

The Blame-Free Organization

THE IMPORTANCE OF REDUCING MEDICATION ERRORS in our hospitals and other healthcare settings hardly needs to be restated. The cost of errors is in the billions of dollars each year and the cost to life is devastating. However, until doctors, pharmacists, nurses, and all other healthcare professionals feel confident that their reporting will remain anonymous and blame-free, and will result in actual change, we may never get to the "zero-error" goal we strive to attain.

Organizational change, from a punitive and judgmental environment to one that is just and blame-free, is critical to ensuring that staff is comfortable reporting medication errors. Unfortunately, according to the Agency for Healthcare Research and Quality (AHRQ), this organizational change has been very slow in coming. (1)

JUST CULTURE

The term *just culture* has been used to define a system with a "non-punitive" or a "blame-free" work environment. It is a term that defines an organization that has established a well-functioning reporting and tracking system to identify processes and behavioral risks that can cause medication errors. This information is then used as the basis for valuable lessons learned and the catalyst for changing this information into action.

Many hospitals state that they are well on their way to achieving a just culture, but the responses from staff do not support this response. (2) The AHRQ Survey found that 65% of staff surveyed worry that mistakes they make are kept in their personnel file; 54% say that when an event is reported it feels like the person is being written up, not the problem; 53% of staff do not feel free to question the decisions or actions of those with more authority; and 50% feel like mistakes are held against them.

Ten Steps to a Just Culture

To achieve a just culture, organizational and behavioral change must occur, including these 10 steps (2):

1. Hospital leadership creates a culture where safety is the primary value.

2. Hospital leadership makes known that sacrificing safety to achieve secondary goals such as productivity and efficiency will not be tolerated.
3. Managers demonstrate that safety is a primary value and practice this in everyday decisions.
4. All staff demonstrates that safety is a sustained primary value, not one that can be reprioritized based on competing demands.
5. Hospital leadership determines what constitutes human error, at-risk behavior, and reckless behavior.
6. Hospital leadership uses system redesign to reduce the risk of human error caused by faulty systems and processes.
7. Hospital leadership manages staff who display at-risk behaviors, shortcuts, or "work-arounds."
8. Hospital leadership acts to ensure that staff who engage in reckless behavior that is intentional, substantial, unjustifiable, and blameworthy, are managed through remedial or disciplinary actions.
9. Hospital leadership develops an effective method for reporting and tracking patient safety information.
10. Hospital leadership creates long-term system remedies, not short-term fixes, and designs reliable systems to prevent errors.

In a just culture, staff is encouraged to report errors and close calls or "near misses" in a timely and factual manner. One essential part of the just culture is an easily accessible, user-friendly, anonymous reporting system. Many hospitals rely on paper forms to report an error and many have converted to a computerized reporting system. Whatever the mechanism, the system should gather data that include the reporter's perceived cause of the problem. Without information about the underlying cause of risk and error, the report holds little value for management to act on and improve safety. (3)

In a just culture, staff must feel that they will not be held liable, nor be the victim of retribution when they report errors. Anonymity, if desired, is essential to obtaining reports that may indicate risks within the department or within the department staff. Fifty- percent of respondents to an AHRQ survey admitted that they did not report risks or errors because they feared that it would be held against them. (3)

In a just culture, hospital leadership and management must be willing to open up about potential risks and errors that have occurred and what actions have been taken to prevent these from happening again. By telling fact-based stories, staff is made aware of how easily an error can occur and changes that have taken place in response. Staff members then feel as though their reporting has led to positive change.

Lastly, in a just culture, hospital and departmental leadership must act upon the reported information and seek long-term solutions rather than short-term, quick-fixes. One study showed that in 93% of the cases studied, nurses used whatever means possible to complete a task, rather than seeking out the underlying cause. (4) Hospitals and other healthcare facilities should devote resources and use trained staff to analyze and work toward achievable and sustainable solutions.

Implementing a Just Culture

- Create a reporting environment where staff members are not fearful of liability or retribution.
- Create a culture where once staff members report an error, they can expect quick and timely feedback from management about what has been done to prevent the error from happening in the future.
- Encourage staff to report faulty systems, especially those that have resulted in dangerous short cuts or work-arounds.
- Inspire and sustain change by telling fact-based stories to illustrate how easily errors can occur. This will help staff understand, remember, and accept the information.
- Develop a comprehensive system for reporting and tracking actual and potential errors.
- Set up systems to analyze and solve problems/systems that lead to errors. These include root cause analysis, failure mode and effect analysis, and rapid process improvement teams.
- Include front-line staff in root cause analysis teams, failure mode and effect analysis, or rapid process improvement teams.
- Refer to outside sources, including the Institute for Safe Medication Practices newsletters, for information about safety issues that have occurred at other healthcare institutions to proactively address and rectify potential errors.

BOTTOM LINE

Work to ensure a just culture by creating a factual and anonymous reporting environment where staff members are comfortable identifying near misses and errors with the goal of re-designing systems to prevent failures in the future.

References

1. Agency for Healthcare Research and Quality. *2012 user comparative database report. Hospital survey on patient safety culture.* Agency for Healthcare Research and Quality. http://www. ahrq.gov/qual/hospsurvey12.

2. ISMP medication safety alert! *Acute Care.* May 17, 2012;17(10).

3. ISMP medication safety alert! Acute Care, July 17, 2012; 17(14).

4. Tucker AL, Edmondson AC. Why hospitals don't learn from failures: organizational and psychological dynamics that inhibit system change. *California Management Review.* Winter 2003; 45(2): 55–72.

CHAPTER 22

Raising the Bar

THE USE OF TECHNOLOGY HAS been shown to reduce medication errors at every stage of the medication use process: prescribing, dispensing, administrating, and monitoring. (1) This technology includes electronic medical records (EMRs), computerized physician order entry (CPOE), barcode medication administration (BCMA), "smart" infusion pumps, automated dispensing cabinets (ADCs), and others. When properly used, the implementation of healthcare technology can reduce errors and improve the quality of care; however, there may be unanticipated risks with its use that should not be ignored.

BARCODE MEDICATION ADMINISTRATION

Barcode medication administration is common in hospitals today. Barcode technology is used at the bedside for patient identification, medication verification, and electronic documentation of dose administration, and is known to decrease medication errors. In a recent process-improvement project in a small Magnet-designated New England hospital, clinical nurse specialists met with experts in pharmacy, information technology, and patient safety to address medication administration safety. This collaborative effort led to a sustained bedside medication scan rate of greater than 97% and a medication error reduction from 2.89 errors per 10,000 doses before implementation of electronic medication administration record to a rate of 1.48 errors per 10,000 doses. (2)

Not all hospitals have demonstrated sustained and successful barcode medication administration practices. Barcode errors can occur for several reasons. For example:

- The nurse may not scan the barcode on the patient's wristband. The patient may not have a wristband or the information on the wristband may be inaccurate. The nurse may find it more efficient to bypass the scan. Or, a barcode scanner may not be available.
- The barcode information on the medication package may be wrong. The barcode may alert the nurse that the medication is wrong, but the nurse may override the alert and administer the medication anyway.

Barcoding in hospitals crosses over multiple disciplines and services and when used appropriately can help prevent serious errors; however, bypassing safety systems and overriding alerts can lead to fatal mistakes.

SMART PUMPS

Intravenous medication infusion pumps or "smart pumps" are another form of healthcare technology that has proven to reduce medication errors. (3) These pumps have built-in safety features such as computers to control the flow of intravenous (IV) fluids and medications, dose calculations, free-flow protection, occlusion alerts, and tamper-resistance for patient-controlled analgesia. These pumps also may provide drug libraries, volume and rate calculations, dose limits, soft and hard alerts, quality improvement reports, clinical advisories, and bolus dose limits. Advanced models include wireless connectivity to other components of the medication administration record and medication safety system.

Medication errors related to smart pumps include improper set-up procedures, such as incorrect entry of the drug, dose, or frequency. Many smart pumps can be preprogrammed for specific medications through the use of drop-down menus with choices for dosages, dose limits, and timing of administration; however, simply hitting the wrong key can result in the selection of the wrong drug or wrong dose.

NOT SO "SMART" PUMPS

A patient in the ICU was given argatroban infusing at a rate of 2mcg/kg/min, using an infusion pump. The ICU nurse programmed the pump to ensure proper dosing, volume, and rate. Later that evening, the patient was transferred to the general medical floor. The floor did not have the same "smart" infusion pump used in the ICU, so the floor nurse had to use the pump she had available. This pump did not have capability to infuse the medication using mcg/kg/min, so she had to calculate the dose in ml/hr. and programmed the pump herself. Needless to say, this complex mathematical equation led to a programing error and the patient was given the wrong dose.

Recognizing that there are many factors that can contribute to infusion errors, the reality is that the technology put into place to prevent errors like this failed, and that technology, in and of itself, does not guarantee patient safety.

AUTOMATED DISPENSING CABINETS (ADCS)

Automated dispensing cabinets (ADCs) are computerized drug storage cabinets that allow medication and other supplies to be stored and dispensed near the point of care, while controlling and tracking distribution. (4) ADCs can provide the nurse with near total access to medications needed in patient care areas, and decrease the delivery time from the pharmacy. ADCs help ensure greater control of the charge capture for medications and may decrease medication error rate. Expanded ADC software provides clinician support for patient safety, machine-readable barcodes for restocking and medication selection, integration into automated refilling systems, drug safety alerts, and decision support when selecting medications and the capacity to link with tele-pharmacy operations for after-hours drug verification and distribution. (4) ADCs also support the Joint Commission medication management standard requiring pharmacist review and approval of all new medications before they are administered to the patient.

Several potential safety hazards are associated with the use of ADCs. These include stocking errors (wrong drug or dosage), diversion of narcotics and other high-alert medications, and staff conditioning that leads them to expect that the same drug/dose will be placed in the same section or drawer each time they access the ADC.

The Institute for Safe Medication Practices has published guidelines for the safe use of ADCs (4), including stocking, pharmacist reviews, location of ADCs, security, inventory, configuration, and processes for overriding, transporting drugs to the bedside, and returning unused drugs.

PREVENTING THE PITFALLS OF HEALTHCARE TECHNOLOGY

- Plan appropriately, train adequately, and allow plenty of practice time before implementing any new health information technology. (5)
- Consider the system usability requirements and the capability of the staff . Is it user-friendly?
- Involve physicians, pharmacists, and nursing staff in the implementation phase to ensure complete buy-in of all technology.
- Consider the system compatibility with the other system in place at your hospital. Proper selection of a system is crucial to success.
- Consider the resources available at your hospital. Phase in different components of these systems over time if necessary.
- Train staff appropriately, including float staff, locum tenens, contract nurses, residents, and new employees.
- Evaluate the impact the new technology will have on workflow and identify potential problems the new systems may cause. Allow time for the staff to meet to reevaluate the new system and the impact it is having on workflow and patient care.
- Do a site visit or phone interview with a current user of the system you are considering. Identify strengths and weaknesses of the new system.

- Anticipate and plan for downtime, having a back up plan when the technology fails or is down for software upgrades, maintenance, power outages, or user error.
- Identify all areas of the hospital that will be impacted by the new technology. If new infusion pumps being used in the ICU may eventually make their way to the floor, make sure staff members throughout the hospital are trained.
- Systematically review overrides and identify work-arounds to determine and eliminate sources of noncompliance.
- Investigate patterns of overrides and discrepancies between stocking, medication inventory, and patient care.
- Identify and address any barriers that arise when the system interferes with workflow or does not perform as described.
- Audit, report, and fix any medication safety issues that occur due to new systems and technology.

BOTTOM LINE

New technologies will provide safeguards; however, they do not guarantee a reduction in medication errors. Do not abandon critical thinking and basic medication administration techniques when prescribing, dispensing, and administering medications.

References

1. Bates DW, Cohen M, Leape LL, et al. Reducing the frequency of errors in medicine using information technology. *J Am Med Inform Assoc.* 2001 Jul-Aug;8(4):299–308.
2. Richardson B, Bromirski B, Hayden A. Implementing a safe and reliable process for medication administration. *Clin Nurse Spec.* 2012 May-Jun;26(3):169–176. doi: 10.1097/NUR.0b013e 3182503fbe.
3. Wilson K, Sullivan M. Preventing medication errors with smart infusion technology. *Am J Health Syst Pharm.* 2004;61(2):177-183.
4. Institute for Safe Medication Practices. http://www.ismp.org. Accessed November 24, 2012.
5. Rausch M. The role of technology in reducing medication errors. *Key Considerations for Health Care Organizations. April 2008; 1–6.*

CHAPTER 23

Deadly Drug Name Mix-Ups

ZANTAC OR XANAX, ZYRTEC OR Zyprexa, PLATINOL OR PATANOL? Many brand name and generic names look alike when written or sound alike when spoken. Simply selecting the wrong drug from the computer drop down menu, writing illegibly, or speaking unclearly can result in the wrong drug being prescribed, leading to catastrophic consequences.

In 2001, the Joint Commission issued a sentinel event alert targeting look-alike/sound-alike (LA/SA) drug names. It identified the need for practitioners and healthcare organizations to be aware of confusing drug names and the impact they had on causing deadly medication errors. The Joint Commission published a list of LA/SA drug names that they believed posed a significant threat. Today, Joint Commission-accredited hospitals maintain a unique list of LA/SA drug names and implement strategies to prevent medication errors from drug name confusion.

The Institute for Safe Medical Practices (ISMP) promotes the use of "Tall-Man" lettering. This is the practice of writing part of a drug's name in upper case letters to draw the eye to specific parts of the drug name and help distinguish look-alike or sound-alike drugs from one another. Tall-Man lettering may be used in hospital computer systems, medication bins, automated dispensing machines, prescription labels, and drug product labels.

The Food and Drug Administration (FDA) and ISMP published a list of recommended Tall-Man letters for look-alike drugs, which includes, but is not limited to:

acetaZOLAMIDE vs. acetoHEXAMIDE

buPROPion vs. busPIRone

chlorproMAZINE vs. chlorproPAMIDE

clomiPHENE vs. clomiPRAMINE

cycloSERINE vs. cycloSPORINE

DAUNOrubicin vs. DOXOrubicin

DOBUTamine vs. DOPamine

hydrALAZINE vs. hydrOXYzine

TOLAZamide vs. TOLBUTamide

vinBLAStine vs. vinCRIStine

In addition to the above list, certain medications have contributed to a high number of medication mix-ups:

- Insulin products such as Novlolin, Novolog, Novolin 70/30, with similar names, strengths and concentrations ratios, have led to hypoglycemia or poor diabetes control.
- Ambisone (amphotericin B liposomal), Abelcet (amphotericin B lipid complex), Amphocin, Fungizone (amphotericin B desoxycholate, conventional amphotericin B) mix-ups have led to dosing errors due to the higher doses of lipid products than conventional products. Confusion may result in respiratory arrest, renal failure and sometimes-fatal adverse events.
- Vinblastine and vincristine mix-ups have led to fatalities when patients were given vincristine at a vinblastine dose.
- Tramadol, trazodone, toradol similar-name mix-ups have led to a decrease in pain control or change in psychiatric symptoms.
- Hydroxyzine, hydralazine, hydrochlorothiazide similar-name mix-ups have led to sedation, hypotension, or other serious adverse events.
- Celebrex, cerebyx, celexa mix-ups have resulted in a decline in mental status or lack of pain or seizure control.

Healthcare organizations have put numerous strategies into place to prevent LA/SA mix-ups. Implementing computerized physician order-entry systems and barcode medication administration systems helps to prevent LA/SA errors. When writing orders, including both the brand and generic name on the prescription, and requiring the printing of the drug names and dosages, helps distinguish one medication from another. Many pharmacies and clinics now store problem medications in separate locations or in different color bins with "Look-Alike/Sound-Alike" stickers affixed to the bins. They also use boldface or color differentiation to reduce confusion on labels, computer screens, automated dispensing devices, and medication administration records.

IS IT ETOPOSIDE OR ETODOLAC?

The inpatient oncology pharmacist reported a near miss. She had received a new order for etoposide injection. This drug is used for the treatment of testicular cancer and small-cell lung cancer. As she was reviewing the medication order, the pharmacist noted that the drug was not prescribed by an oncologist, but by a new resident in the outpatient general medicine clinic. She also found that the patient did not have cancer at all! The pharmacist contacted the resident for clarification. The resident stated that he did not want etoposide injection for this patient, but etodolac, a non-steroidal anti-inflammatory for the patient's arthritis pain. He must have picked the wrong drug in the computer by mistake since etoposide was just under etodolac in the computer drug menu. The error never reached the patient but shows how easily dangerous errors can happen with look-alike and sound-alike drugs.

STAY VIGILANT—KNOW YOUR LOOK-ALIKE/ SOUND-ALIKE DRUGS

- Maintain awareness of look-alike and sound-alike drug names. Refer to your hospital's unique LA/SA drug list and make recommendations for additions to the list as appropriate. (1,2)
- Ensure that professional staff is aware of the hospital's LA/SA drug list. Just knowing that there are LA/SA drug names that cause errors may help prevent them.
- Avoid abbreviating drug names. MSO4 or MgSO4? Morphine sulfate or magnesium sulfate?
- With problematic name pairs, reduce the potential for confusion by using both the brand and generic drug name on the prescription: Toradol (ketorolac), Ultram (tramadol).
- Specify the dosage form, drug strength, and complete directions on the prescription. This will help pharmacists distinguish between look-alike and sound-alike drug products.
- Whenever possible, include the purpose of the medication on the prescription. Most products with look-alike or sound-alike drug names are for different purposes. This also helps patients and caregivers know what the drug is for once they get home.
- Alert patients and caregivers to the potential for a mix-up with problematic drug names. Tell patients to insist on pharmacist counseling at the prescription counter to make sure the medication name, use, directions, and side effects match what you have told them.
- Use verbal or telephone orders only when absolutely necessary. Include the drug's intended purpose to ensure clarity. Ask the nurse or pharmacist to read back all verbal/phone orders to you to ensure accuracy.
- Never order chemotherapy verbally.
- Report near misses and errors resulting from look-alike and sound-alike medications to your hospital's medication safety personnel or the FDA MedWatch program at www.fda.gov.

BOTTOM LINE

- Healthcare practitioners and organizations should be aware of the role look-alike and sound-alike drug names play in dangerous medication errors. Providers should make changes, as recommended above, to prevent these errors from happening to their patients.

References

1. ISMP. What's in a name? Ways to prevent dispensing errors linked to name confusion. *ISMP Medication Safety Alert!* 7(12) June 12,2002.
2. JCAHO. *Sentinel Event Alert.* Issue 19, May 2002.

CHAPTER 24

Dangerous Drug Interactions

RUG INTERACTIONS AFFECT MILLIONS of people each year and are a significant cause of medication errors leading to emergency room visits and
hospital admissions. (1) Drug interactions are defined as the pharmacologic or clinical response to the administration of a drug combination different
from that anticipated from the known effects of the two agents when given alone.
(2) These include interactions between two prescription drugs, interactions between
a prescription and an over-the-counter (OTC) drug, or interactions between a
prescription drug and an herbal product or nutritional supplement. Interactions
may also occur when certain drugs are taken with certain foods. Many of these
interactions are unknown, unpredictable, and unavoidable; however, many other
interactions are well documented, probable and entirely preventable.

The risk of drug interactions increases with the number of prescription drugs taken
(polypharmacy). Drug interactions may also increase with the number of OTCs,
herbals, supplements, or natural medications taken. Drug interactions may lead
to patient injury, hospital admission, prolonged stay, disease progression, and
increased healthcare costs. (3)

While many drug interactions can be prevented, it is unrealistic to expect clinicians
to memorize thousands of drug–drug interactions and their clinical significance.
This is especially difficult with new drugs constantly coming to market. Computer systems have been designed to alert providers of potentially dangerous drug
interactions; however, computer systems also may alert providers to insignificant
or minor interactions. This leads to "alert fatigue" and the possibility that major
notifications are overridden and dangerous interactions occur.

COMMON PRESCRIPTION DRUG INTERACTIONS

1. Lisinopril taken with spironolactone: The combination of an ace inhibitor
   with a potassium sparing diuretic can lead to hyperkalemia. This is also true
   when an ace inhibitor is combined with a potassium supplement or potassium
   containing salt substitutes.
2. Fluoroquinolones, sulfa drugs, and macrolide antibiotics (erythromycin, clarithromycin, azithromycin, and others) taken with warfarin may lead to an
   increased risk of bleeding.

3. Simvastatin taken with erythromycin, ketoconazole (Nizoral), iraconazole (Sporanox), clarithromycin (Biaxin), telithromycin (Ketek), cyclosporine (Sandimmune),nefazodone (Serzone), boceprevir (Victrelis), telaprevir (Incivek), voriconazole (Vfend), posaconazole (Noxafil), and HIV protease inhibitors such as indinavir (Crixivan) and ritonavir (Norvir) could increase the levels of simvastatin in the body and increase the risk of muscle toxicity from simvastatin.

COMMON PRESCRIPTION AND OVER-THE-COUNTER (OTC) DRUG INTERACTIONS

1. OTC NSAIDS (ibuprofen, naproxen, aspirin, and others) taken with warfarin may increase the risk of bleeding.
2. OTC H2 receptor antagonists (cimetidine and other acid reducers) taken with citalopram may lead to a prolongation of the QT interval.
3. OTC antihistamines and night-time sleep aids such as diphenhydramine taken with benzodiazepines, narcotics, tricyclic antidepressants, certain antihypertensive and other medications with anticholinergic properties, may lead to excessive sedation.

FORBIDDEN FRUIT

The interaction between certain prescription drugs and grapefruit juice has been well-documented since the 1990s; however, just recently many other drugs have been added to this list.(4,5) The updated list below is not all-inclusive:

1. Anti-cancer agents (such as crizotinib, cyclophosphamide, dasatinib, everolimus, and many others) and grapefruit juice may lead to myelotoxicity or torsade de pointes.
2. Anti-infective agents (such as erythromycin, praziquantel, primaquine, and others) and grapefruit juice may lead to myelotoxicity, torsade de pointe, and other dangerous reactions.
3. Anti-lipemic agents (such as atorvastatin, lovastatin, simvastatin) and grapefruit juice may lead to rhabdomyolysis.
4. Cardiovascular agents (such as amiodarone, cilostazol, clopidogrel, ticagrelor, verapamil, and many others) and grapefruit juice may lead to torsade de pointes, hypotension, peripheral edema, and complete heart block.
5. Central nervous system agents (such as buspirone, dextromethorphan, fentanyl, ketamine, methadone, quetiapine, ziprasidone, and others) and grapefruit juice may lead to hallucinations, somnolence, sedation, respiratory depression, and torsade de pointes.
6. Immunosuppressant agents (such as cyclosporine, sirolimus, everolimus, tacrolimus, and others) and grapefruit juice may lead to nephrotoxicity or myelotoxicity.

7. Urinary tract agents (such as darifenacin, solifenacin, tamsulosin, and others) and grapefruit juice may lead to urinary retention, constipation, postural hypotension, and in the case of solifenacin, may lead to torsade de pointes.

COMMON SENSE STRATEGIES FOR PREVENTING DRUG INTERACTIONS

- Never automatically override computerized clinical decision support tools that alert for potential drug interactions, especially if these are major or severe.
- Instruct patients to inform you of all of the over-the-counter medications, natural products, herbal remedies, nutritional supplements, vitamins, etc., that they are taking and have them add these to their medication list.
- Consider the use of concurrent drug therapies or over-the-counter agents as the cause of unusual or unanticipated reactions to a medication.
- Consider the use of concurrent drug therapies or over-the-counter agents as the cause of unusual or unanticipated lab results, i.e., hyperkalemia or hyponatremia.
- Instruct patients to avoid eating grapefruit or pomelos or drinking grapefruit juice when taking certain medications. Supply patients with a current list of medications that interact with grapefruit juice.
- Make sure patients are aware of the potential for an adverse reaction with grapefruit juice and the type of reaction that may occur. Instruct patients what to do if a reaction occurs.
- Use alternative agents that do not interact with grapefruit juice if there is a possibility that this may happen.
- Instruct patients to ask their pharmacists about potential drug–drug, drug–OTC, and drug–food interactions.

BOTTOM LINE

- Clinicians should be aware of drug–drug, drug–OTC, and drug–food interactions and require patients to notify them of any new prescription drugs or over the counter agents they are taking.

References

1. Juurlink DA, Mamdani M, Kopp A, Laupacis A, Redelmeier, DA. Drug-drug interactions among elderly patients hospitalized for drug toxicity. *JAMA*. 2003 Apr 2;289(13):1652-1658.
2. Tatro DS. *Drug interaction facts*. St. Louis, MO: JB Lippincott Co., 1992.
3. Penzak SR. *Drug interactions*. Bethesda, MD: National Institutes of Health, 2010.
4. Rabin RC. Grapefruit is a culprit in more drug reactions. *New York Times*. December 17, 2012. D6. http://well.blogs.nytimes.com/2012/12/17/grapefruit-is-a-culprit-in-more-drug-reactions/?_php=true&_type=blogs&_r=0
5. Bailey DG, Dresser G, Arnold JM. Grapefruit-medication interactions: forbidden fruit or avoidable consequences? *CMAJ*. 2013 Mar 5;185(4):309-16. doi: 10.1503/cmaj.120951. Epub 2012 Nov 26.

CHAPTER 25

Caution: Other Serious Side Effects May Occur

ADVERSE DRUG REACTIONS (ADRs), SIDE effects, and allergies have been reported with just about every drug class. These reactions are generally due to the pharmacologic nature of the drug or unforeseen or unknown patient characteristics, and are generally considered to be non-preventable. ADRs include allergic or hypersensitivity reactions and can manifest as rash, swelling, or difficulty breathing. ADRs also can be a direct pharmacologic result of the drug itself, such as hypotension, dizziness, and lethargy with an antihypertensive drug. Other ADRs have no known cause (idiosyncratic) and are simply unique to that individual patient.

ADRs may be mild, such as upset stomach or rash, and result in the discontinuation of the drug. Other ADRs may be severe such as anaphylaxis, rhabdomyolisis, or Steven-Johnson Syndrome, and result in hospitalization. An ADR may have happened in the past, like a childhood reaction to penicillin, or it may be new one, like a stuffy nose with sildenafil. Regardless when the reaction occurred, it should be accurately documented in the patient's medical record to prevent it from happening again.

Predicting who will have an adverse drug reaction is difficult. Although older age, severity of illness, multiple comorbidities, and polypharmacy may be associated with adverse reactions, no real cause and effect exists. Medication type is not a reliable indicator either. Medications found to be problematic include antibiotics, analgesics, cardiovascular drugs, sedatives, antineoplastics, and anticoagulants. However, many other drugs cause adverse reactions such as antipsychotics, antidiabetics, antidepressants, antihistamines, and antiemetics. (1) Additionally, since the Food and Drug Administration (FDA) trials are limited for new drugs, these reactions may not even be evident for many years after the drug is on the market and has been taken by thousands of people.

The FDA MedWatch program is a voluntary reporting database for serious adverse drug events or product problems. The FDA uses this database to maintain safety surveillance for all FDA-regulated drug products and devices. Reporting adverse reactions to the FDA is critical to improving the safety profile of a drug and increasing overall patient safety. (2)

CITALOPRAM ALERT!

In August 2011 and then again in March 2012, the FDA alerted providers of deadly heart rhythm abnormalities about the use of citalopram. This alert was based on post-marketing adverse reaction reports received by the FDA of QT interval prolongation and torsade de pointes in patients taking citalopram at doses greater than 40mg per day.

Celexa, the brand name for citalopram, was first brought to market in 1998 and has been taken successfully by thousands, if not millions of people since then. However, based on newly documented reports from providers, 14 years later there is a major change to the prescribing and dosing recommendations for this drug. Doses are now significantly lower to no more than 20mg in patients over 60 years old and no more than 40mg in patients overall.

Additionally, the FDA identified other drugs that if take concurrently, could potentially increase the concentration of citalopram and increase the risk of QT prolongation. Lastly, recommendations include ECG and electrolyte monitoring to identify patients who may be at risk for heart rhythm abnormalities and discontinuation of the drug if the QTc persistently exceeds 500msec.

Voluntary reporting by providers to the FDA have led to the revisions of citalopram labeling and directly affected the overall safety of this drug.

AVOID ADVERSE DRUG REACTIONS

- Possibly reduce the severity or even eliminate some adverse drug reactions by initiating and following different drug administration procedures. For example, suggest that the patient take the medication with meals to prevent stomach upset or take it at bedtime to avoid drowsiness and fatigue.
- Document adverse drug reactions, allergies, and side effects in the patient's medical record.
- Report all serious adverse drug reactions to the FDA MedWatch system, including those resulting in hospitalization.
- Report to the FDA MedWatch system, all adverse events related to new drug therapies (on the market fewer than three years). This alerts the FDA to adverse events that may not have surfaced during the clinical trials.
- Educate patients on the adverse reactions, allergies, and side effects of new medications. Ensure that they know who to call or what to do in the event they experience an adverse reaction.

- Encourage patients to keep a medication list, including any adverse reactions or allergies they have had in the past.
- Ask patients to update you on any new allergies or ADRs that may have occurred since their last visit. Also ask patients to remind you of any historical reactions or allergies; be certain they are listed in the medical record.
- Be mindful that certain populations, including the elderly or the young, may be especially susceptible to adverse drug reactions and that adjustments to therapy may be necessary.
- Educate patients and caregivers in advance about common adverse reactions, i.e., upset stomach or drowsiness, and advise them what to do if they experience these reactions. Simply taking the medication with a meal or at bedtime may be enough to prevent these.
- Encourage patients to purchase a medical alert bracelet or necklace if there are severe allergies or reactions.
- Refer patients, especially those prone to adverse events, to specialized clinics for follow-up care. These may include pharmacist- or nurse-run clinics for anticoagulation, pain management, mental health, substance abuse, chronic disease management, heart failure, hepatitis C, and others.
- If available, ask that a pharmacist counsel your patient prior to hospital discharge. This will help ensure all new medications and potential adverse reactions are reviewed.
- If available, utilize computer technology to alert providers of any adverse reactions or allergies that the patient has experienced in the past.
- Take the time to educate your patients about their medication therapy using the NUTS method: Name of the drug, what it is Used for, how to Take it safely, and what Side effects to expect. This will increase your patients' knowledge of their medication therapy and will help increase the trust they have in you.

BOTTOM LINE

Adverse drug reactions, side effects, and allergies are generally considered to be non-preventable adverse events; however, these may be greatly reduced by diligent reporting, patient education, and use of the resources currently available to you.

References

1. Agency for Healthcare Research and Quality. Reducing and preventing adverse drug events to decrease hospital costs. *Research in Action.* March 2001: 1-10.
2. MedWatch reporting form at: www.fda.gov

CHAPTER 26

Risky Business!

RECENT STUDIES (1) HAVE LINKED inappropriate prescription drug use in elderly patients with:

1. Adverse drug events contributing to unnecessary hospitalizations;
2. Increased length of hospital stay;
3. Increased duration of illness;
4. Nursing home/rehab placement; and
5. Falls that lead to physical and functional decline.

As a result, the Centers for Medicare and Medicaid Services (CMS) has included the Use of High Risk Medications in the Elderly in its Clinical Quality Measures (CQM) for 2014.

CQM Measure: Percentage of patients 66 years of age and older who were ordered high-risk medications.

Two rates are being reported:

1. Percentage of patients who were ordered at least one high-risk medication; and
2. Percentage of patients who were ordered at least two different high-risk medications.

Domain: Patient Safety

WHY THE CONCERN?

Prescribing high-risk medications in patients over the age of 65 is dangerous, especially when safe and effective alternatives are available. According to the Agency for Healthcare Research and Quality (AHRQ), inappropriate prescribing of medications in the elderly is an important quality of care issue. Past studies in ambulatory and long-term care settings have shown that 27% of adverse drug events in primary care and 42% in long-term care were preventable, with most problems occurring with prescribing and monitoring medications. (2,3) A study of the 2000/2001 Medical Expenditure Panel Survey revealed that the total estimated healthcare expenditures related to the use of potentially inappropriate medications in the elderly was $7.2 billion. (4)

In 2012, the American Geriatrics Society published the updated criteria for potentially inappropriate medication use in older adults (Beers criteria). The updated criteria focuses on 53 medications or medication classes divided into three categories:

1. Potentially inappropriate medications and classes to avoid in older adults;
2. Potentially inappropriate medications and classes to avoid in older adults with certain diseases and syndromes that the drugs listed can exacerbate; and
3. Medications to be used with caution in older adults. (5)

Of note, the Beers list of potentially inappropriate medications and classes to avoid in older adults includes new additions: megestrol, glyburide, and sliding-scale insulin. New inclusions to the list of potentially inappropriate medications and classes to avoid in older adults with certain diseases and syndromes that the drugs listed can exacerbate are thiazolidinediones or glitazones with heart failure, acetylcholinesterase inhibitors with history of syncope, and selective serotonin reuptake inhibitors with falls and fractures. Lastly, included in the list of medications to be used with caution in older adults are two new antithrombotics: dabigatran and prasugrel. These two agents bear a caution of increased bleeding risk for adults 75 years or older.

According to the Centers for Medicare and Medicaid (CMS) and the National Committee for Quality Assurance (NCQA) the drugs listed in the table below should be avoided or used with caution in the senior population. These drugs are considered to have a high risk of side effects, limited efficacy, or can exacerbate existing conditions. (6)

LESS IS MORE!

- Providers may contact the pharmacist for recommendations for alternative agents to high-risk medications. In some instances, lower doses or a safer non-pharmacological therapy may be substituted for the use of a high-risk medication.
- Incorporating Beers criteria into computerized order entry systems (CPOE) can ensure providers are alerted of high-risk medications during the prescribing process.
- Healthcare systems have already started to implement "hard stops" for high-risk medications prescribed for elderly patients. These prescriptions are being rejected back to providers for alternative therapies or additional documentation.
- Providers should pay attention to the "flags" or other pharmacy notifications alerting them to a high-risk medication. Address these "flags" appropriately

High-Risk Medications in the Elderly

Therapeutic Class	Medication Name
Antianxiety	• meprobamate • aspirin-meprobamate
Antiemetic	• trimethobenzamide • scopolamine
Analgesic	• ketorolac • acetaminophen-diphenhydramine • diphenhydramine-magnesium salicylate
Antihistamines	• APAP/dextromethorphan/diphenhydramine • APAP/diphenhydramine/phenylephrine • APAP/diphenhydramine/pseudoephedrine • acetaminophen-diphenhydramine • codeine/phenylephrine/promethazine • diphenhydramine-pseudoephedrine • dexchlorpheniramine/guaifenesin/PSE • dexchlorpheniramine-pseudoephedrine • dexchlorpheniramine/dextromethorphan/PSE • dexchlorpheniramine/methscopolamine/PSE • diphenhydramine-magnesium salicylate • diphenhydramine/hydrocodone/phenylephrine • atropine/CPM/hyoscyamine/PE/PPA/scolpolamine • dexachlorpheniramine/hydrocodone/phenylephrine • promethazine • diphenhydramine • hydroxyzine hydrochloride • diphenhydramine-tripelennamine • diphenhydramine-phenylephrine • cyproheptadine • dextromethorphan-promethazine • codeine-promethazine • phenylephrine-promethazine • dexaclropheniramine • tripelennamine • hydroxyzine pamoate • carbetapentane/diphenhydramine/ phenylephrine
Antipsychotics, typical	• thioridazine • mesoridazine
Amphetamines	• dexmethylphetamine • pemoline • dexmethylphenidate • amphetamine-dextroamphetamine • methylphenidate • phentermine • methamphetamine • benzphetamine • phendimetrazine • diethylpropion
Barbiturates	• amobarbital • secobarbital • pentobarbital • butabarbital • mephobarbital • phenobarbital
Long-acting benzodiazepines	• chlordiazepoxide • flurazepam • amitriptyline-chlordiazepoxide • diazepam • chlordiazepoxide-clidinium
Calcium channel blockers	• nifedipine—short acting only
GI antispasmodics	• propantheline • dicyclomine
Belladonna alkaloids	• belladonna/ergotamine/phenobarbital • atropine/hyoscyamine/PB/scopolamine • butabarbital/hycosyamine/phenzopyridine • digestive enzymes/hyoscyamine/phenyltoloxamine • belladonna/caffeine/ergotamine/pentobarbital • atropine/CPM/hyoscyamine/PE?scoplamine • hyoscyamine/methenam/m-blue/phenyl salicyl • atropine • atropine–difenoxin • atropine-diphenoxylate • hyosycamine • belladonna • atropine-edrophonium • hyosycamine-phenobarbital

Skeletal muscle relaxants	• ASA /caffeine/orphenadrine • ASA/carisoprodol/codeine • aspirin – meprobamate • methocarbamol • aspirin-methocarbamol • aspirin-carisoprodol • cyclobenzaprine • orphenadrine • carisprodol • chlorzoxazone • metaxalone
Oral estrogen	• esterified estrogen-methyltestosterone • conjugated estrogen • estropipate • esterified estrogen • conjugated estrogen-medroxyprogesterone
Oral hypoglycemics	• chlorpropamide
Narcotics	• ASA/caffeine/propoxyphene • meperidine • propoxyphene napsylate • pentazocine • acetaminophen-pentazocine • belladonna-opium • acetaminophen-propoxyphene • meperidine-promethazine • naloxone-pentazocine • propoxyphene hydrochloride
Vasodilators	• cyclandelate • ergot mesyloid • isoxsuprine • dipyridamole-short acting only
Others	• methyltestosterone • thyroid desiccated • nitrofurantoin macrocrytals • nitrofurantoin • nitrofurantoin macrocrystals-monohydrate

and completely to ensure all healthcare providers are aware of the rationale for use of this particular medication.

• Several drugs have recently undergone FDA labeling changes to include dose warnings for patients over the age of 65. As patients age, providers need to adapt the dose the patient is currently taking with new dosing/age recommendations.

• Providers must be notified of any changes to existing medications or additions of new medications where Beers Criteria will apply.

• Minimizing the use of high-risk medications in the elderly will help reduce unnecessary harm and the associated costs of care.

BOTTOM LINE

Studies have shown that high-risk medications continue to be prescribed for vulnerable elderly adults. Providers should be aware of these high-risk medications and use alternative agents when appropriate. If a high-risk drug is determined to be the only agent available to effectively treat the patient, then close monitoring for adverse drug events should be done to prevent unnecessary patient harm.

References

1. Agency for Healthcare Research and Quality. Use of high-risk medication in the elderly. Agency for Healthcare Research and Quality. http://www.qualitymeasures.ahrq.gov. Accessed July 11, 2013.

2. Gurwitz JH, Field TS, Harrold LR, et al. Incidence and preventability of adverse drug events among older persons in the ambulatory setting. *JAMA*. 2003 Mar 5;289(9):1107–1116.

3. Gurwitz JH, Field TS, Judge J, et al. The incidence of adverse drug events in two large academic long-term care facilities. *Am J Med*. 2005 Mar;118(3):251–258.

4. Fu AZ, Jiang JZ, Reeves, JH et al. Potentially inappropriate medication use and healthcare expenditures in the US community-dwelling elderly. *Med Care*. 2007 May;45(5):472-476.

5. American Geriatrics Society 2012 Beers Criteria Update Expert Panel. American Geriatrics Society updated Beers Criteria for potentially inappropriate medication use in older adults. *J Am Geriatr Soc*. 2012 Apr;60(4):616–631. doi: 10.1111/j.1532-5415.2012.03923.x. Epub 2012 Feb 29.

6. National Committee for Quality Assurance. High risk medications. National Committee for Quality Assurance. http://www.ncqa.org. Accessed July 11, 2013.

CHAPTER 27

You Aren't as Unique as You Think!

MEDICATION ERRORS THAT RESULT from improper patient identification can happen during patient registration, prescribing of medications, blood draws, infusions, order transcription, dispensing of medications, administering of medications, monitoring effects, the discharge process, and any other point in the patient's hospitalization. (1)

One of the most common "wrong patient" errors happens when a nurse administers a medication meant for someone else. However, wrong-patient errors can happen when the prescriber enters the order on the wrong patient, or when the pharmacist mis-transcribes a phone order and fills the prescription for the wrong patient. Wrong-patient errors happen when the nurse confuses two patients with similar sounding names or when the test results are mixed up and one patient gets results meant for another. Nurses have been discouraged from using verbal confirmation of the patient's name such as "You're Mr. Jones, right?" as a substitute for verifying the patient's full name and checking the wristband.

Wrong-patient errors can be compounded when two patients have the same or similar last names. It is fairly common to see two patients on the same nursing unit with the same last name. According to the U.S. Census Bureau, the 10 most common last names in October 2012 were (3):

1. Smith
2. Johnson
3. Williams
4. Brown
5. Jones
6. Miller
7. Davis
8. Garcia
9. Rodriguez
10. Wilson

TWO PATIENT IDENTIFIERS

The Joint Commission has established a National Patient Safety Goal to ensure accurate verification of each patient at all stages of the medication use process. This goal requires that healthcare providers use at least two patient identifiers (not the room number or patient location) when providing care, treatment, or services. The reason for this safety goal is to 1) reliably identify the individual as the person for whom the service or treatment is intended and 2) match the service or treatment to that individual. Acceptable identifiers may be the patient's name, identification number, telephone number, or other person-specific identifier. (1)

CORRECT PATIENT IDENTIFICATION

- Use at least two identifiers (full name, date of birth, address, telephone number) to verify the patient's identity. Be sure to include Jr. and Sr. designations. (2)
- Do not identify patients using passive agreement ("You're Mrs. Jones, right?").
- Utilize the time-out process for correct identification; include the patient in the verification when possible. The time-out is standardized pre-procedure verification process involving the immediate members of the procedure team who actively communicate and verify the correct patient, correct site and correct procedure.
- Implement processes to identify patients who lack proper identification. This can include alternate means of identification such as state ID, veterans ID, school ID, date of birth, social security number, home address, and others.
- Educate patients regarding the identification processes used in your hospital or office, or the process they may experience during a procedure. Let them know that they may be asked to identify themselves several times by several different people, and that this is for their protection and safety, yet guarantees their privacy.
- Encourage patients and their families to actively participate in the identification process.
- Be sure patients know that each healthcare provider who comes into contact with them (pharmacist, lab tech, radiologist, nurse, therapist, etc.) must correctly identify himself or herself to them.
- Implement computer provider order entry (CPOE) systems and barcoding systems to decrease patient identification errors. If CPOE is already in place, limit the selection of patients to only those patients on your panel.
- If your facility allows the use of verbal orders, consider using a preprinted template order pad that prompts for all necessary information (e.g., patient's full name, medical record number or patient identification number, date of birth, etc.).

- Confirm all verbal orders by reading the order back to the provider.
- Ensure the medication being prescribed makes sense for that particular patient given the clinical circumstances.
- Implement processes for an independent double check of a patient when prescribing selected high-alert drugs (i.e., chemotherapy, insulin).
- Inform patients of the name of and reason for the drug, and encourage patients to ask questions if something does not seem right.
- Employ barcode verification of the patient's wristband prior to medication administration.
- Implement strategies to accurately verify patients with common names. This may include using the patient's social security number, date of birth, or address. However, patients with the same last name may live at the same address, including parents and adult children as well as siblings. Many hospitals and individual providers have started to take a picture, which is kept in the medical record to assist with verification.
- Implement strategies, like patient labels or prominent notation, that will alert staff about name confusion and trigger them to identify the patient by alternative means.

BOTTOM LINE

Wrong-patient errors can happen at any time, anywhere in the medication use process. Patients should be accurately identified to ensure the individual is the person for whom the service or treatment is intended and to match the service or treatment to that individual.

References

1. The Joint Commission. National patient safety goals. The Joint Commission. http://www.jointcommission.org/assets/1/6/OBS_NPSG_Chapter_2014.pdf. Accessed November 12, 2012.
2. Institute for Safe Medication Practices. Oops, sorry, wrong patient! Applying the JC "two-identifier" rule beyond the patient's room. *ISMP Medication Safety Alert*, June 3, 2004.
3. U. S. Census Bureau. Genealogy data: frequently occurring surnames from Census 2000. U. S. Census Bureau. http://www.census.gov/genealogy/www/freqnames2k.html. Accessed October 28, 2012.

CHAPTER 28

Get to the Root
of the Problem

WHEN A MEDICATION ERROR OCCURS, it disrupts the lives of the patient, physician, pharmacist, nurse, and all other staff involved. Whether the error resulted in a fatal outcome or was a close call, errors are taken seriously and personally and need to be addressed swiftly and with respect and professionalism. It is at this time that the root cause analysis process comes into use.

Root cause analysis (RCA) is a valuable tool for improving medication safety and future patient outcomes. The goal of root cause analysis it to learn as much as we can from situations that do not turn out as we had hoped or come too close for comfort. RCA can help us learn the truth about why an event happened and then help us apply what we learned constructively, so we can do something better in the future and ultimately prevent adverse events and close calls from happening again. (1)

The "root cause" is the most basic reason that a situation did not turn out as we had planned or expected. There may be more than one root cause to any situation, but most often the root cause is a known or unknown *system vulnerability*. Human weakness is almost never a root cause.

Root causes are those that can reasonably be identified and are those over which management has control. (2) Snow storms, power outages, and floods are not controlled by management. Neither are "operator error," or "equipment failure." These "causes" are general classifications and are not specific enough for management to make effective changes. Root causes need to be targeted and actionable before management can take steps to prevent the event from happening again.

Root causes are those for which effective recommendations can be generated. (2) Improving adherence to policies, improved training, and hiring more staff are not considered effective recommendations for addressing root causes. Recommendations should always address the specific root cause identified during the team's investigation by going directly to the source of the problem. Creating systems and process that will not allow an error to occur is the most effective strategy for preventing adverse events from happening in the future.

THE RCA TEAM APPROACH

When an error occurs, a Root Cause Analysis Team may be convened. This team is tasked with reviewing the event and the factors leading to the event. This is a multi-disciplinary team made up of a team leader (facilitator) and staff (including front-line) who are familiar with the day-to-day tasks involved in the event.

An experienced facilitator who can keep the team on track and produce expected results in a time-efficient and cost-effective manner is charged with leading the RCA team. It is not productive to keep valuable resources tied up indefinitely searching for the root cause and subsequent solutions. The team pinpoints and focuses on the specific causes of the event and what, if changed, would stop the event from happening again. The more precise the team can be in identifying the root cause, the easier and more successful it will be in recommending solutions and preventing a recurrence.

There are several basic tools relevant to root cause analysis teams. These include:

1. Data Collection—This should begin as soon as possible and be as complete as possible.
2. Causal Factor Charting—A flow diagram should be developed that describes what happened in the time leading up to and during the event.
3. Root Cause Mapping—This is a decision tree that helps focus the process on *why* a particular causal factor exists or occurred. Asking the "5 Whys" will help investigators target the specific root cause of the event.
4. Recommendations, Implementation and Sustaining Improvement—The RCA team is tasked with creating realistic, achievable recommendations for preventing the recurrence of the event.

NO KNOWN ALLERGIES

A 35-year-old white male experienced a cardiac arrest while undergoing elective arthroscopy on his right knee as a day surgery patient. The patient had no history of prior medical problems, and "NKA" (no known allergies) was listed in his chart.

The anesthesiologist reported that the patient appeared to react to the cefazolin that was administered intraoperatively. The reaction to the cefazolin caused the patient to become hypotensive and arrest.

A root cause analysis team was convened immediately to review the circumstances leading to this event. This team was made up of staff who were knowledgeable of the systems and processes in the operating room and who were capable of analyzing the situation. The team toured the area and interviewed the staff involved in order to obtain complete and current information.

The team met to construct the first draft of a process flow diagram, charting the steps leading to the actual event. Additional information was filled in as the investigation proceeded.

The RCA team determined that the patient was admitted to the day surgery center on the date of occurrence. The admission staff noted "NKA" in the patient's chart and did not ask if there were any new allergies to add. The patient was sent to the pre-op area where the anesthesiologist reviewed the patient's chart. The physician noted the term "NKA" and assumed that the information was up-to-date. He administered cefazolin intravenously to the patient. The patient began to experience hypotension and shortness of breath and despite resuscitative efforts, died. It was later discovered that the patient had experienced shortness of breath several months earlier after taking cephalexin for an upper respiratory infection; however, there was no documentation of this in the patient's surgical records.

After the flow-charting was finalized, the team created a root cause map. By listing the causal factors and asking the "5 Whys," the team was able to identify one causal factor and determine one root cause statement:

1. Causal Factor: Due to the notation of "NKA" or no known allergies in the patient's chart, the admissions clerk did not ask if the patient had any new allergies to report.
2. Root Cause Statement: Due to the notation of "NKA" or no known allergies in the patient's chart, the anesthesiologist administered a drug the patient was allergic to.

The team then created the following recommendations to avoid similar occurrences in the future:

1. Admissions clerks to ask and verify current allergy information, including asking if there are any new allergies, on every patient on the day of surgery. This verification will be documented by the admissions clerk (including date) in the patient's chart. No patient will be allowed into the pre-op area without this information in the chart.
2. Anesthesiologists to verify that there is current allergy information in the patient's chart before administering any medication. This verification must be signed and dated by the administering anesthesiologist.

To ensure recommendations would be enacted, the head of surgery, head of nursing, and manager of the admissions clerks reviewed and agreed to the recommendations and met to plan for their enactment. To ensure sustainment, the manager of the admissions clerks would run monthly reports to ensure appropriate allergy documentation. To ensure allergy verification by anesthesiologists, the head of surgery incorporated this verification into the "time out" checklist for the procedure. Any deviation from either of these two practices would result in disciplinary action.

EFFECTIVE ROOT CAUSE ANALYSIS STRATEGIES

- Provide "just-in-time" RCA team training as part of the first team meeting to review basic process improvement tools.
- Select team members who are interested in finding solutions to the event, and who have the expertise, commitment, and time to participate in team meetings.
- Enlist the active support of top management in the RCA process. This will ensure that you have management buy-in as well as their perspective, including any limitations you may not be aware of.
- Let the team leader lead the meeting and let the recorder record the minutes. Include a computer/systems-literate member on each team.
- Create a clear and concise problem statement. Always involve a specific cause and effect and refrain from individual blame or accusations.
- Give teams a general timeline at the first meeting and try to stay as close to this timeline as possible to ensure the RCA is done in a timely manner.
- Don't waste team meeting time trying to create a perfect flowchart. These can be fine-tuned after the meeting.
- Apply wise time-management strategies during meetings. Use agendas, stay focused and on task, ensure full team participation, and use strategies to bring teams to full consensus quickly.
- Interview department heads or service directors who are likely to be involved in implementing the actions of the RCA to seek opinions and experiences and to learn about what has already been tried and how to avoid potential obstacles. Don't blindside these colleagues—it's not fair or professional.
- Be cognizant of costs involved in your recommendations. Expensive fixes will require some homework and cost justification analysis before presentation to the management team.
- Have the RCA team report to management and cover "what we found," the "recommendations," and "what is needed from management." This will provide the team with recognition from the executive management team as well as clear communication/understanding about what additional follow-up work needs to be done.
- The RCA team often is not responsible for implementing the team recommendations; however, someone must be responsible for ensuring the recommendations are implemented and that measures are in place to monitor the effectiveness and sustainability of these recommendations.

- Organizations must ensure that recommendations are tracked and reported in an ongoing and systematic manner. This could include monthly inspections, tracers, environment of care rounds, and others.
- Share the successes of the team at staff meetings, in newsletter articles, at town hall meetings, etc.
- Tell your own stories and make it safe for others to tell theirs.
- Don't try to "solve world hunger" with your RCA team. Create a "lessons learned" chart with additional issues that need management attention at a later time.

BOTTOM LINE

Root cause analysis provides a mechanism to identify not only *what* and how an event happened, but also *why* it happened. Only when we are able to determine why an error or close call occurred are we be able to create specific, focused workable actions to prevent that error from happening in the future.

References

1. Veterans Administration National Center for Patient Safety. Root cause analysis. Veterans Administration National Center for Patient Safety. http://www.patientsafety.va.gov/professionals/onthejob/rca.asp.
2. Rooney JJ, Vanden Heuvel LN. Root cause analysis for beginners. *Quality Progress*, July 2004: 45-53.

CHAPTER 29

The Lean Transformation

Toyota created Lean Six Sigma manufacturing principles in post-World War II Japan to reduce production waste, unnecessary downtime, and costly mistakes. Those same principles can be instrumental in transforming systems in hospitals today. (1) Lean techniques are designed to decrease medication errors, eliminate wasteful processes and procedures, and increase value and quality.

MUDA

According to Taiichi Ohno, the Toyota executive who created lean thinking, "LEAN is the relentless pursuit of the elimination of waste." Waste is described by the word *muda*. *Muda* is evident in mistakes that require correction, production of goods without demand, or inventories of stockpiled supplies. Waste includes unnecessary steps within a process, as well as unnecessary movement of employees or employees standing idle waiting for an activity to be completed. (2)

According to the American Society of Health-System Pharmacists, waste in the medication use system includes: (3)

- Waste of Correction: medication errors, adverse drug events, hospital-acquired infections;
- Waste of Overproduction: extra oral medications or IVs returned to pharmacy;
- Waste of Material/Information Movement: "missed doses," unnecessary STATs;
- Waste of Motion: poor departmental layout resulting in unnecessary steps and actions;
- Waste of Waiting: workload and productivity imbalance;
- Waste of Inventory: excess stock/low inventory turns;
- Waste of Processing: multiple systems/duplication of entries; and
- Waste of Creativity: not using the knowledge and experience of staff to solve problems.

Lean transformation is a process in which the efficiency, cost, and quality of a process are improved by the application of lean principles, notably the reduction of waste. By applying Lean principles to the medication use systems, processes will be streamlined and improved, and medication errors will be reduced. (3)

To be successful, Lean improvements require eight basic steps: (4)

133

1. Ensure management commitment and buy-in;
2. Perform just-in-time training in lean concepts for employees (during first meeting);
3. Identify the key process to be addressed;
4. Flowchart the current state of the process;
5. Identify the metrics that will provide measurement of success;
6. Flowchart the future state of the process (what should happen);
7. Perform a gap analysis between the current state and the future state and develop recommendation to achieve the future state; and
- Implement the future state recommendation.

TRANSFORMING CARE

The executive leadership team in a large managed care organization identified the need to increase patient throughput in a busy dermatology clinic. Currently there was a four-month wait time for a new patient appointment. A Lean process improvement team was chartered to address this issue. The Lean team was selected by an executive steering committee and was comprised of individuals experienced with the dermatology consulting and scheduling process.

The first step for the team was to clearly define the project as it related to patient throughput in the dermatology clinic. The team created an initial project charter with a detailed/limited scope, timeline and communication plan. It also included input from the organization, the clinic staff and the patients themselves. It was found that there were numerous complaints from patients regarding the wait time and that many patients had to seek treatment outside of the organization leading to higher costs.

The team began to measure baseline data associated with the dermatology consult/scheduling process. This included a detailed process map and baseline metrics as well as time studies associated with each step in the process. The team then had to analyze the data and identify any potential root causes of delays. What the team found were several time-consuming, redundant steps in the process leading to referrals being delayed, reworked or lost. Once these causes were identified, the team developed and implemented potential solutions in order to improve the process. These solutions included new, streamlined referral forms for providers and a new scheduling process.

The last step was to control the process by developing standard operating procedures and control systems to ensure any/all new processes put into place would sustain over the long run. Following the implementation of the new consults, measurements showed a decrease in dermatology wait time to 2 months. This resulted in a cost savings to the organization and an improvement in patient satisfaction and care.

THE SKEPTICS

So why the skepticism and why has Lean taken so long to catch on in healthcare?

It may be due in part to the fact that healthcare professionals are well-educated and by nature focused on doing the best at all times. If they encounter a problem they quickly come up with a solution. (1) Healthcare professionals are too busy to discuss the overall processes on their floors and then come up with global solutions; however, most of the providers are inherent problem solvers and with the strategy of "thinking Lean," they are able to step back, think about the problem in the context of the entire workflow, and generally come up with a workable solution.

THE LEAN SOLUTION

- Lean process improvement is characterized by recognition of the wasteful process, comparison to an ideal lean state, and implementation of systemic changes.
- Lean transformation is not a quick-fix QI project. Lean transformation requires a change in management and staff awareness of ways to continuously improve day-to-day workflow processes.
- There may be some resistance to lean thinking, as some of the recommended changes may be counter-intuitive or go against "the way we have always done it." Change management and continued support by department managers are important for lean transformations to occur.
- If automation is implemented, there should be department "super-users" and appropriately trained staff, as this may change the workflow.
- Staff will feel discomfort as they transition to new processes. Anticipate this. The tendency to resort to old habits should be expected and managed.
- Leadership support is key to making the lean project succeed. This includes departmental leadership as well as leadership from other affected departments (medicine, nursing, pharmacy, lab, etc.)
- Communicate, communicate, and communicate.

BOTTOM LINE

Healthcare institutions are being asked to do more with their existing staff. To meet these demands institutions can employ lean thinking, which will eliminate waste, decrease errors, improve efficiency, and provide value to patients.

References

1. Boston Consulting Group. Lean health care: lower costs, better results. Boston Consulting Group. http://knowledge.wharton.upenn.edu. Accessed March 22, 2013.

2. Womack J, Jones D. *Lean thinking: Banish waste and create wealth in your corporation.* New York: Simon and Schuster, 2003.

3. American Society of Health-System Pharmacists. Applying LEAN to the medication use process: issues for pharmacy. American Society of Health-System Pharmacists. https://www.ashp.org/DocLibrary/Policy/QII/ApplyingLEAN_Flyer.pdf

4. Diorio L, Thomas D. Lean concepts and pharmacy. LDT Health Solutions Inc. ldthealthsolutions.com/_articles/LeanConceptsAndPharmacy.pdf. Accessed March 22, 2013.

CHAPTER 30

5S—The Visual Workplace

O NE OF THE EASIEST YET most powerful lean tools is 5S. 5S helps identify and eliminate waste and reduce errors in a process or environment. 5S creates a "visual workplace" where waste and abnormal conditions are readily apparent to anyone who works in that area. It stresses "a place for everything and everything in its place." The 5S process creates a workplace that is clean, well-organized and standardized, resulting in an easier, less confusing, less error-prone, less stressful work environment.

5S stands for:

1. **Sort:** Eliminate unnecessary items and tasks. Get rid of what you don't need and "red tag" any items that are questionable.
2. **Straighten:** Effectively organize what you need to keep. Eliminate the need to "search for stuff" and make the environment "visual" through the use of obvious triggers or "Kanbans."
3. **Shine:** Thoroughly clean and shine the work area. Staff will take pride in an area that is clean and clutter-free.
4. **Standardize:** Develop standardized processes that apply to everyone who works in that area.
5. **Sustain:** Make the 5S processes part of the everyday routine and schedule routine review teams to develop action plans when necessary.

The goal of the 5S process is to identify and eliminate waste. Waste is defined as:

- Defects—medication errors, readmissions or hospital acquired conditions;
- Overproduction—large batches of materials and supplies when not necessary;
- Waiting—beds, clinics, paper work, tests, labs, etc.;
- Not utilizing employee's knowledge and creativity (non-optimized resources;
- Transport—incorrect floor layout, patient flow;
- Inventory/Inspection—redundant activities, excessive waste of time/manpower;
- Motion—searching for medications, information; and
- Extra processing—Fragmented workflow, unnecessary approvals.

The Institute for Healthcare Improvement (IHI) states that there is growing agreement "among healthcare leaders that Lean principles can reduce the waste that is pervasive in the U.S. healthcare system. Adoption of Lean management strategies—while not a simple task—can help healthcare organizations improve processes and outcomes, reduce cost and increase satisfaction among patients, providers and staff." (1)

5S—MANAGING CHAOS

Several medication errors had been reported due to prescriptions being filled with the wrong quantity from the pharmacy processing area. As a result, patients were complaining about not getting the right number of pain pills and there was a loss of productivity as the technicians and pharmacists had to take time to research, verify, and refill these orders.

One look in the processing area and it was easy to see why these mistakes were being made. The area was cluttered, disorganized, overcrowded, and appeared to lack standardized processes. This chaotic mess was causing a lack of efficiency, decreased productivity, and poor morale among the staff. The technicians who worked there often complained of being cramped and bumping into each other while trying to get prescriptions filled. The director of pharmacy believed the pharmacy processing area (and the employees who worked there) would benefit from a 5S reorganization initiative.

A team was formed that included the lead technician, the computer systems technician, and a staff technician. A quality improvement pharmacist led the team. The team met one hour a week for six weeks and members were taught basic lean techniques such as process flow mapping, spaghetti diagrams, checklists, and time studies.

The goals of the 5S initiative were to improve workflow by reorganizing the workspace, improve efficiency, decrease rework, and get the medications to the patients quickly and safely.

The first thing the team did was to Sort (5S #1), which meant they removed all old or unnecessary items from the workspace. This included removing all boxes of old prescription records and relocating them to external storage site, removing old equipment that was no longer being used, removing all unnecessary items and supplies, and returning unused or overstock inventory to supplier. The team then set in order (5S #2) the medication shelves to maximize space and organization.

A spaghetti diagram was used to determine daily workflow patterns. The team found that the majority of work was being done in one area; the other side of the space was hardly used. Since this was a very small space to begin with, the team decided that they needed to redesign the workspace to maximize workflow. Internal redesign was accomplished over a weekend and new countertops were created to better fit the room design. Computers were added, printers were moved, and a new desk was installed for the lead technician. Housekeeping was then called in to clean and shine (5S #3) the floors and counter tops.

To standardize (5S #4) the processes, new procedures were created for processing controlled substance returns and new storage areas were created for storing these returns until destruction. A new workflow process standardized work from the filling tech to the checking pharmacist to the technician packaging the prescription to be mailed to the patient.

To sustain (5S #5) the orderliness and cleanliness in the area, the team takes turns sweeping and doing daily maintenance. There is also a three-month inspection along with other routine checks.

YOU NEVER KNOW UNTIL YOU ASK!

During one of the early 5S team meetings, one of the technicians said it would be really nice if they had a robot in the processing area. "This way" she stated, "we could get all of the work done in half the time." Medication filling robotic equipment is expensive, and on a limited hospital budget, this request seemed highly unlikely, but the team wrote it on their "wish list" and proceeded to present the 5S results to the executive leadership team. The project had been successful, there was a place for everything and everything was in its place, workspace was now open and no one was bumping into each other, the shelves were reorganized to maximize efficiency, and returned medications were being processed in a timely and efficient manner.

Before the presentation concluded, the executive leadership team inquired about the robot and asked what it could do to increase efficiency in the pharmacy. The technicians on the team had done their homework and were ready for this question. They had calculated that the robot could fill in one and one-half hours what it was taking three techs to do in an eight-hour shift. They also determined that once they had finished their daily work in the processing area, they could be productive in other areas of the pharmacy. Lastly, the robot could continue to process orders for other areas of the pharmacy after the work in the processing area was done. Needless to say, the efficiencies and subsequent cost savings impressed the executive team. They agreed that the robot would be a great addition to the pharmacy and added it to the budget for the following year!

TIPS FOR A SUCCESSFUL 5S PROJECT

- Sustain all organizational efforts. This is by far the most critical step in the 5S process. Without active, consistent and supported sustainment, the project is doomed to fail.

- Ensure leadership support. This includes providing time/additional staff to cover meetings, actively participating in selection of projects, utilizing "positional power" to ensure support from ancillary departments, providing funding for meals on the day of project, entertaining requests for funding if project necessitates it, and all other supervisory and leadership functions. This is active leadership support, not just "lip service" to yet another quality improvement initiative.
- Select a focused and attainable project.
- Select a team that is aware of the issues impacting this project and have the expertise to suggest/implement solutions.
- Perform a direct observation of the affected area.
- Select a meeting time that meets everyone's needs and work with managers to free up staff to attend meetings.
- Train the 5S team in 5S/lean principles.
- Take lots of pictures, both before and after. Pictures tell a story that words cannot possibly describe.
- Communicate, communicate, communicate with front-line staff, managers, administrators, and all other impacted workers. Communicate at each step of the process to provide feedback to the staff and kudos for the 5S team working on the project.
- Pick a day for the project when everyone can attend and be relieved of other duties until the project is complete.
- Provide (good) food during the project day.
- Plan all aspects of each 5S step completely and methodically.
- Set up ancillary services (housekeeping, data systems, record storage, etc.) and confirm that they will be there to assist prior to or during the 5S initiative.
- Be sure to have sufficient supplies, including brooms, buckets, rags, cleaner, tape, scissors, label makers, post it notes, markers, etc.
- Utilize triggers or "Kanbans" to assist with visual inventory management. This will help create situational awareness so the staff knows when they are ahead, behind, or on schedule, or if there is something wrong.
- Standardize the processes and educate staff on new process requirements. Then educate again. Print article in department newsletters and post pictures on bulletin boards. Create a Power Point presentation for use at staff meetings and for the department director to show his or her supervisor.
- Sustain all organizational efforts. This is by far the most critical step in the 5S process. Without active, consistent and supported sustainment the project is doomed to fail.
- Reward the team with kudos and recognition.
- Make 5S a part of the leadership strategy, including front-line staff, managers, supervisors, and all other members of the workforce.

BOTTOM LINE

5S is an easy yet powerful lean tool that enables department leaders to maximize productivity with their existing staff.

Reference

1. Womack, JP, Byrne A, Flume O, et al. *Going lean in health care.* Institute for Healthcare Improvement. Cambridge, MA: IHI, 2005.

Promote Prevention

Medical science has proven time and again that when the resources are provided, great progress in the treatment, cure, and prevention of disease can occur.

MICHAEL J. FOX

CHAPTER 31

ABCs of HBP

CARDIOVASCULAR DISEASE IS THE LEADING cause of death in the United States. Each day, 2,200 people die from cardiovascular disease. Every year, more than 2 million Americans have a heart attack or stoke and more than 800,000 of these people die. (1) Medical costs and productivity losses approach $450 billion annually and these costs are expected to triple over the next two decades if present trends continue. (2)

In an effort to significantly reduce the number of Americans with cardiovascular disease, the Centers for Medicare and Medicaid Services (CMS) has included Controlling High Blood Pressure as one of the Clinical Quality Measures for 2014. This measure includes the percentage of patients 18–85 years of age who had a diagnosis of hypertension and whose bleed pressure was adequately controlled (<140/90mmHg) during the measurement period.

To help achieve this goal and lower the risk of cardiovascular disease in the United States, the U. S. Department of Health and Human Services, along with other federal agencies and private-sector organizations, have launched the Million Hearts initiative. The goal of this initiative is to prevent 1 million heart attacks and strokes in the United States over the next five years. (3)

The Million Hearts initiative seeks to achieve this goal by: (3)

1. Empowering Americans to make healthy choices, such as quitting smoking and reducing sodium and trans fat consumption, and
2. Improving care by targeting the ABCS of high blood pressure: Aspirin, Blood pressure control, Cholesterol management and Smoking cessation.

Improving the management of the ABCS can prevent more deaths than other clinical preventive services. (4) It is estimated that less than half of the people who have ischemic heart disease take daily aspirin; less than half who have hypertension have it adequately controlled; only a third who have hyperlipidemia have adequate treatment; and less than a quarter of smokers who try to quit get counseling or medication. As a result, more than 100 million people—half of American adults—smoke or have uncontrolled high blood pressure or cholesterol. Many have more than one risk factor. It is estimated that utilizing the ABCS interventions could save more than 100,000 lives a year. (4)

The goals of the Million Hearts initiative align well with the CMS Clinical Quality Measures (CQMs) and the adult recommended core measures for Stage 2 Meaningful Use. (3)

1. Million Hearts: Aspirin Use

Meaningful Use: Ischemic Vascular Disease (IVD)—Use of aspirin or another antithrombotic.

Measure: Percentage of patients ages 18 years or older with IVD with documented use of aspirin or other antithrombotic.

2. Million Hearts: Blood Pressure Control

Meaningful Use: Hypertension (HTN)—Controlling high blood pressure

Measure: Percentage of patients ages 18–85 years who had a diagnosis of HTN and whose blood pressure was adequately controlled (<140/90) during the measurement year.

3. Million Hearts: Cholesterol Screening and Control

Meaningful Use: Preventive Care and Screening—Cholesterol—fasting low density lipoprotein (LDL) test performed AND risk-stratified fasting LDL

Measure: Percentage of patients ages 20—79 years whose risk factors have been assessed and a fasting LDL test has been performed AND who had a fasting LDL test performed and whose risk- stratified fasting LDL is at or below the recommended LDL goal.

4. Million Hearts: Smoking Cessation

Meaningful Use: Preventive Care and Screening—Tobacco Use
Measure: Percentage of patients ages 18 years and older who were screened about tobacco use one or more times within 24 months and who received cessation-counseling intervention if identified as a tobacco user.

CONTROLLING HIGH BLOOD PRESSURE

- Distribute patient education materials regarding cardiovascular disease, cholesterol management, and smoking cessation by going to: http://millionhearts.hhs.gov/resources.html
- Provide information to patients about smoking cessation programs and help them enroll before they leave the office.
- Provide patients with a specific diet plan and measurable weight loss goals. Provide them with a method to monitor and track their weight loss and ask

for a routine update regarding their progress via secure email, electronic messaging, etc.

- Provide patients with a blood pressure cuff and have them monitor their blood pressure routinely. Ask them to report back to you if they have any higher-than-anticipated readings.
- Identify patient-specific risk factors or lifestyle habits that contribute to elevated lipid levels. Have patients work with a dietician if necessary to eliminate or substitute high-fat foods.
- Use the community pharmacist to promote medication adherence and provide assistance with obtaining free or low-cost medications.
- Use the team-based approach to cardiovascular disease management. Involve advanced practice nurses, pharmacists, dieticians, and community health partners to maximize use of resources available locally, regionally, and nationally.

Bottom Line

Reducing the incidence of cardiovascular disease and preventing 1 million heart attacks and strokes by 2017 will require commitment from providers, pharmacists, nurses, community-based services, and the patient themselves. However, with initiatives such as the Million Hearts initiative, this should be a realistic goal.

References

1. Frieden Tr, Berwick, DM. The "million hearts" initiative—preventing heart attacks and strokes. *N Engl J Med.* 2011 Sep 29;365(13):e27. doi: 10.1056/NEJMp1110421. Epub 2011 Sep 13.
2. Heidenreich PA, Trogdon JG, Khavjou OA, et al. Forecasting the future of cardiovascular disease in the United States: a policy statement from the American Heart Association. *Circulation.* 2011 Mar 1;123(8):933-944. doi: 10.1161/CIR.0b013e31820a55f5. Epub 2011 Jan 24.
3. U. S. Department of Health and Human Services. Million Hearts Initiative. http://www.million hearts.hhs.gov
4. Farley TA, Dalal MA, Mostashari F, Frieden TR. Deaths preventable in the U. S. by improvements in use of clinical preventive services. *Am J Prev Med.* 2010 Jun;38(6):600-609. doi: 10.1016/j.amepre.2010.02.016.

CHAPTER 32

Up in Smoke

TOBACCO USE IS THE NUMBER one preventable cause of morbidity and mortality in the world today. (1) In the United States, tobacco use adds $96 billion in healthcare costs each year. In 2010, 45 million U.S. adults smoked and approximately one-half of them will die of a tobacco-related disease, losing an average of 10 years of life. (1) Smoking is directly responsible for 1 in 6 of all deaths in the United States each year and is the major cause of heart attacks, strokes, lung cancer, chronic bronchitis, and emphysema. (2)

Approximately 20 million of the 70 million young adults in the United States under the age of 18 smoke cigarettes. About 5 million of the 20 million will eventually die due to smoking-related diseases. Cigarette companies spend more than $3 billion each year in advertising campaigns promoting cigarettes. This advertising is so effective that is lures 3,000 new young smokers every day. (2)

Nicotine, which is just as addictive as cocaine and heroin, is added to every cigarette. The average smoker takes approximately 10 puffs per cigarette. Multiply that by 20 cigarettes per pack and the average one-pack per day smoker takes 200 puffs of highly addictive nicotine daily. Upon inhalation, nicotine causes a pleasurable sensation in the brain and reduces stress in just seven seconds. (2) The initial euphoria is quickly replaced by a powerful craving for more nicotine and the addiction starts. In fact, nicotine withdrawal begins within two hours after the last cigarette. If smokers do not get the nicotine fix, they suffer withdrawal symptoms including irritability, restlessness, insomnia, nausea, and sweats.

The Centers for Medicare and Medicaid Services (CMS) has included Preventive Care and Screening: Tobacco Use: Screening and Cessation Intervention in the Clinical Quality Measures for 2014. The measure includes the percentage of patients aged 18 years and older who were screened for tobacco use one or more times within 24 months and who received cessation counseling intervention if identified as a tobacco user.

In addition to being a Clinical Quality Measure, CMS has also included tobacco use in the Stage 2 Core Objectives for Eligible Professionals.

Objective: Record smoking status for patients 13 years old and older.

Stage 1: More than 50% of all unique patients 13 years old and older seen by the EP have smoking status recorded as structured data.

Stage 2: More than 80% of all unique patients 13 years old and older seen by the EP have smoking status recorded as structured data.

Smoking cessation can drastically reduce the risk of suffering from tobacco-related illness and disease. It is also one of the most cost-effective strategies in healthcare. Tobacco use is a chronic, relapsing disorder that often starts in childhood and endures throughout adult life. Treating tobacco addiction as a chronic disease may require a multi-pronged approach that includes behavioral support (counseling) and medication therapy.

BEHAVIORAL SUPPORT

Smoking cessation may require the smoker to break bad habits as well as break the addiction. By providing counseling, providers can help the smoker break bad habits that lead to tobacco abuse. Brief clinical interventions by primary care providers can help promote smoking cessation; however, there is a strong dose-response between the intensity of tobacco counseling and it effectiveness (3). Primary care clinicians have limited time to address smoking cessation effectively during the routine office visit and can benefit from using available resources and relying on team-based care.

THE "5 A'S" BRIEF COUNSELING MODEL

Using the "5 A's" (Ask, Advise, Assess, Assist and Arrange) can help start the conversation with your patients and lead to smoking cessation.

1. **Ask:** "Do you currently use tobacco?" It is recommended that patients be asked a minimum of three times per year in the primary care setting and once a year in specialty care settings unless they are lifetime non-smokers or quit more than seven years ago. The office staff can help complete this step.
2. **Advise:** This is the physician's role and is key to helping patients quit. The physician should strongly advise the smoker to quit. The message may be more urgent when advising pregnant women.
3. **Assess:** Ask "Are you willing to quit now?" The purpose of this step is to assess readiness to quit; however, a new approach is not to ask if the smoker is ready, but to simply offer treatment. Stating, "Quitting smoking can be difficult, here are some options to help you" may be a more effective approach and lead to greater success. If they are not willing to quit, intervene to increase motivation to quit. Use the 5 R's: Relevance, Risks, Rewards, Roadblocks, and Repetition.
4. 4. Assist: Provide appropriate treatment, including medication and counseling.

5. **Arrange:** Connect to resources in the community or health system and provide a follow-up plan.

Proactive, private, convenient, and free counseling is available in the United States. Resources include:

1-800- QUIT-NOW: This is a free telephone support service that can help individuals who want to stop smoking or using tobacco. Callers have access to several types of cessation information and services, including:

- Free support and advice from experienced counselors;
- A personalized quit plan;
- Self-help materials;
- Social support and coping strategies;
- The latest information about cessation medications; and
- Over-the-counter nicotine replacement medications for eligible participants in more than half of U.S. states.

www.becomeanex.org: The EX Plan is a free quit smoking program that helps patients re-learn life without cigarettes. This site shows patients how to deal with the things that trip up people when they try to quit smoking so they will be more prepared to quit and stay tobacco-free.

www.quitnet.com: QuitNet is the world's largest and most comprehensive online quit-smoking service, offering the tools and support patients need to quit and stay tobacco-free.

MEDICATION OPTIONS

Using medications to help quit smoking (nicotine replacement, bupropion, or varenicline) can double the chances of success. (3) Pharmacotherapy can help lessen withdrawal symptoms and suppress the urge to smoke.

Nicotine replacement therapy (NRT) provides nicotine without a cigarette and helps alleviate withdrawal symptoms while the smoker quits. These products include over-the-counter skin patches, gum and lozenges, and well as prescription oral inhalers and nasal sprays. Current FDA labeling warns smokers against the use of multiple nicotine replacement products at the same time; however, U.S. Public Health Service clinical guidelines recommend combining the long-acting patch with the shorter-acting NRT product to maintain an adequate nicotine blood level and have a way to respond to urgent cigarette cravings. (3)

Bupropion is an antidepressant that increases smoking cessation rates independent of its antidepressant properties. It is associated with an increased risk of seizure and therefore is contraindicated in patients with a history of seizures. It may be helpful for patients who are concerned about weight gain post-cessation.

Varenicline is a smoking cessation product that relieves nicotine withdrawal symptoms and blocks the reinforcement of smoking by blocking nicotinic receptors. In 2009, a black box warning was added to varenicline and bupropion labeling due to post-marketing case reports of behavior changes. These behaviors included hostility, agitation, depression, and suicidal thoughts or actions. (4) However, it still remains to be determined if these effects are attributed to the drug or to the withdrawal symptoms themselves.

In 2011, the FDA issued a warning that varenicline may increase the risk of cardiovascular events in patients with cardiovascular disease. (5) Although this risk still remains to be verified, it is up to the provider and the patient to determine if these medications are safe and effective for the patient. Clinicians who prescribe these agents should monitor patients for changes in behavior and mood, especially those patients with a history of mental health issues.

BE SMOKE FREE

- Treat tobacco use as a chronic illness, using multiple treatment modalities to increase the success rate.
- Utilize medication therapy along with behavioral counseling to achieve optimum success.
- Use medication therapy appropriately and maximize its potential before stopping. Always consider patient non-adherence with medication therapy before changing to alternate treatments.
- Limit the use of e-cigarettes until the safety and effectiveness is proven.
- Initiate smoking cessation counseling by using the "5 A's." This brief counseling technique (5-10 minutes) has proven successful.
- Ask for assistance from office staff in "Asking" patients if they currently use tobacco.
- When "Assessing" the readiness to quit, don't ask "Are you willing to quit now?" Rather, offer treatment.
- Use resources available to you as a provider. Fax or use an e-referral to ensure that the patient is contacted by a quit line, rather than relying on the smoker to contact the quit line.
- Ask for back up! Use personnel to help counsel patients and provide follow up. This is especially relevant to the patient-centered medical home model. New "health coaches" are being used to help with patient counseling and monitoring in smoking, weight management, alcohol, and drug abuse.

BOTTOM LINE

- Don't give up! Optimize behavioral support and medication therapy to ensure the highest rate of success.

References

1. Centers for Disease Control and Prevention. Vital signs: current cigarette smoking among adults aged ≥18 Years—United States, 2005–2010. *Morbidity and Mortality Weekly Report,* September 9, 2011 / 60(35);1207–1212.
2. Bruce Algra. Facts about smoking. Bruce Algra Posters. http://www.algra.com. Accessed December 11, 2012.
3. Fiore MC, Jaen CR, et al. *Treating tobacco use and dependence: 2008 update.* Rockville, MD: U.S. Department of Health and Human Services, 2008.
4. Food and Drug Administration. *Public health advisory: FDA requires new boxed warning for the smoking cessation drugs Chantix and Zyban.* Food and Drug Administration. http://www.fda.gov. Accessed December 11, 2012.
5. Food and Drug Administration. *FDA drug safety communication: Chantix (varenicline) may increase the risk of certain cardiovascular adverse events in patients with cardiovascular disease.* Food and Drug Administration. http://www.fda.gov. Accessed December 11, 2012.

CHAPTER 33

Worth the Weight!

APPROXIMATELY ONE-THIRD OF U.S. ADULTS are obese (as defined Body Mass Index of 30 kg/m2 or greater). (1) The American Heart Association has identified obesity as an independent risk factor for coronary heart disease (CHD). Additionally, a number of metabolic changes such as insulin resistance, type 2 diabetes, hyperlipidemia, hypertension, left ventricular hypertrophy, sleep apnea, heart failure, ECG changes, and abdominal obesity are associated with obesity, and may increase the risk of coronary heart disease. (2) Healthcare costs linked to obesity exceed $110 billion annually. (3)

The 2014 Centers for Medicare and Medicaid (CMS) include preventive care and screening of body mass index (BMI) in the Clinical Quality Measures for 2014. This measure includes the percentage of patients ages 18 years and older with a documented BMI during the reporting period AND when the BMI is outside of normal parameters a follow-up plan is documented.

Normal Parameters:

Age 65 years and older BMI ≥ 23 and < 30

Age 18 – 64 years BMI ≥ 18.5 and < 25

Weight loss can help improve or prevent risk factors for CHD by reducing the incidence of diabetes, improving lipid profile, and decreasing blood pressure. (4) It has been shown that even a modest weight loss (5%) can positively impact cardiovascular risk factors. In the Diabetes Prevention Program, a multi-center trial in patients with impaired glucose tolerance, a weight loss of 7% reduced the rate of impaired glucose tolerance to diabetes by 58%. (5)

Despite the recommendations that primary care physicians offer their obese patients advice and counseling regarding weight management, particularly those with known cardiovascular risk factors, clinicians often find that time and effective strategies for addressing weight reduction are both limited. Weight loss should be addressed using a combination of diet, exercise, and behavioral modification. In some patients, pharmacologic treatment or bariatric surgery may be necessary.

DIET

Excess intake of calories and a sedentary lifestyle cause weight gain and obesity. The average adult requires 22 kcal/kg to maintain a kilogram of body weight. The average reduction of 500kcal/day should result in a weight loss of approximately 0.5kg/week (~1 lb week). However, after 3–6 months of dieting, energy expenditure adaptations may diminish ongoing weight loss. (6) The goal of any diet is to reduce energy intake from food. (7)

There are several different types of diets. The choice of diet depends on the degree of obesity and patient preference.

1. **Balanced low-calorie diets**—These diets include foods with adequate nutrients, including protein, carbohydrates, and essential fatty acids, and don't include alcohol, sugar-containing beverages, and most highly concentrated sweets.
2. **Portion-controlled diets**—These diets include the use of individually packaged foods, formula diet drinks, nutrition bars, and pre-packaged meals to maintain 1000–1500 kcal per day.
3. **Low-fat diets**—These diets keep calories from fat below 30% of total calories or 30 grams of fat for each 1000 calories consumed. In a low-fat diet, the decrease in fat should be combined with an increase in healthy carbohydrates (fruits, vegetables, and whole grains).
4. **Low-carbohydrate diets**—Low-carb diets that include 60–130 grams of carbohydrate and very low carbohydrate diets that include 0–60 grams of carbohydrate are popular and may be effective for short-term weight loss. (7) However, saturated fats and unhealthy proteins should be avoided and healthy choices for fat (mono and polyunsaturated) and protein (fish, legumes, nuts, and poultry) should be encouraged.
5. **High protein diets**—This includes diets that are more than 50% protein. The American Heart Association doesn't recommend high-protein diets for weight loss because some of these diets restrict healthful foods that provide essential nutrients and do not provide the variety of foods needed to adequately meet nutritional needs.
6. **Mediterranean diet**—This diet includes a high level of monounsaturated fat; moderate consumption of alcohol (wine); high consumption of vegetables, fruits, legumes, and grains; moderate consumption of milk and dairy products (cheese); and low intake of meat and meat products.

PHARMACOTHERAPY

Along with diet and exercise, drug therapy may be necessary for the treatment of obesity. However, the decision to initiate drug therapy should be carefully evaluated due to the risks versus benefits of weight-loss treatments. (8) Anti-obesity drugs may be useful in patients with a BMI greater than 30kg/m2 or in those with sleep apnea or other comorbid conditions. (9)

1. **Diethylpropion (Tenuate):** FDA approved for short–term use. Decreases appetite and increases the feeling of fullness. May increase blood pressure and heart rate, and may cause insomnia and dizziness.
2. **Locaserin (Belviq):** FDA approved for long-term use. Decreases appetite and increases the feeling of fullness. May cause headache, dizziness, fatigue, nausea, dry mouth, and constipation.
3. **Phentermine (Adipex):** FDA approved for short–term use. Decreases appetite and increases the feeling of fullness. May increase blood pressure and heart rate, and may cause insomnia and dizziness.
4. **Orlistat (Xenical):** FDA approved for long-term use. Works by blocking the absorption of fat. May cause intestinal cramps, gas, diarrhea, oily spotting. Available as an over-the-counter product in reduced strength (Alli).
5. **Phentermine/topiramate extended-release (Qsymia):** FDA approved for long-term use. Decreases appetite and increases the feeling of fullness. May cause increased heart rate, birth defects, tingling of hands and feet, insomnia, dizziness, constipation, and dry mouth.

WATCHING YOUR WEIGHT

- Set realistic goals. A weight loss goal of 5–7% is realistic and beneficial for most patients.
- Pick the diet regimen most suited for your patient. This includes the degree of obesity and patient preference.
- Pick a diet regimen that reduces energy intake below energy expenditure rather than focusing on the macronutrient composition of the diet.
- Behavior modification may be useful in the treatment of obesity and is provided by trained personnel or self-help groups.
- Patients who are overweight (BMI >27kg/m2) or obese (BMI >30kg/m2) should receive counseling on diet, lifestyle, and goals for weight loss.
- Include exercise to increase energy expenditure, especially in the maintenance of long-term weight loss.
- Drug therapy may be a useful adjunct to diet and exercise for obese patients (BMI >30 kg/m2 or BMI >27–30kg/m2 with comorbid conditions).
- Bariatric surgery may be an option for patients with severe obesity that has not responded to other methods of weight loss (diet and exercise with or without drug therapy). This includes patients with a BMI ≥40kg/m2 or BMI ≥35kg/m2 with serious comorbidities.

BOTTOM LINE

In the United States, 34% of adults ages 20 years and older are overweight, 34% are obese, and 6 % are extremely obese. However, fewer than half of obese adults report being advised by their doctors to lose weight. Clinicians must play an active role in educating patients about the serious dangers of obesity and the optimal strategies for losing weight.

References

1. Flegal, KM, Carroll MD, Ogden CL, Curtin LR. Prevalence and trends in obesity among US adults, 1999–2008. *JAMA*. 2010 Jan 20;303(3):235–241. doi: 10.1001/jama.2009.2014. Epub 2010 Jan 13.
2. Eckel RH. Obesity and heart disease: a statement for healthcare professionals from the Nutrition Committee, American Heart Association. *Circulation*. 1997 Nov 4;96(9):3248-50.
3. Finkelstein EA, et. al. National medical spending attributable to overweight and obesity: how much, and who's paying? *Health Aff (Millwood)*. 2003: *Suppl Web Exclusives: W3-219-W3-226.*
4. Klein S, Burke, LE, Bray GA, Blair S, et al. Clinical implications of obesity with specific focus on cardiovascular disease: a statement for professionals from the American Heart Association Council on Nutrition, Physical Activity, and Metabolism: endorsed by the American College of Cardiology Foundation. *Circulation*. 2004 Nov 2;110(18):2952–2967. Epub 2004 Oct 27.
5. Knowler WC, Barrett-Connor E, Fowler SE, et al. Reduction in the incidence of type 2 diabetes with lifestyle intervention or metformin. *N Engl J Med. 2002; 346:393.*
6. Hall KD, Sacks G, Chandramohan D, Chow CC, et al. Quantification of the effect of energy imbalance on bodyweight. *Lancet.* 2011 Aug 27;378(9793):826–837. doi: 10.1016/S0140-6736(11)60812-X.
7. Freedman MR, King J, Kennedy E. Popular diets: a scientific review. *Obes Res.* 2001 Mar; 9 Suppl 1:1S-40S.
8. National Institutes of Health. *The practical guide. Identification, evaluation, and treatment of overweight and obesity in adults.* Washington, DC: NIH, 2000. NIH Publication Number 02-4084
9. Mayo Clinic. Prescription weight loss drugs: Can they help you? The Mayo Clinic. http://www.mayoclinic.com/health/weight-loss-drugs/WT00013. Accessed December 30, 2012.

CHAPTER 34

The Exercise Rx

STRONG SCIENTIFIC EVIDENCE SUGGESTS THAT frequent moderate-to-vigorous exercise plays a significant role in preventing cardiovascular disease, type 2 diabetes, obesity, and some cancers. (1) However, due to today's rapid growth in technology, many people now spend the majority of their workday seated at a computer screen, then spend the remainder of their day at home to playing video games or watching TV. Prolonged sitting and a general lack of physical activity are two major contributing factors to the obesity epidemic in the United States today.

The American College of Sports Medicine is researching why too much daily sitting is so bad for your health. They are finding that too much sitting impairs the body's ability to deposit fat from the blood stream into the body. These constantly elevated blood fats are a risk factor for cardiovascular disease. Additionally, researchers have found that too much sitting during the day impairs the functioning of the body's HDL cholesterol, thus reducing the body's ability to rid itself of arterial plaque. Studies are indicating that moving more during the day, in addition to getting the daily 30 minutes of moderate activity, is necessary to lower the risk of cardiovascular disease and other causes of mortality. (1)

Despite the fact that physicians have been prescribing exercise for many years, patients may find it necessary to have a detailed and comprehensive exercise prescription including realistic physical activities and goals. Simply stating "You need to drop 20 pounds" may not be enough information for your patient to be successful.

The Centers for Disease Control and Prevention (CDC) states that physical activity is anything that gets the body moving. There are two types of physical activity that patients should do each week to improve their health: aerobic and muscle strengthening. (2) This combination helps to maintain or improve cardiorespiratory and muscular fitness and overall health and function. (1)

A complete physical activity action plan for adults should include (2):

Plan A:

Two hours and 30 minutes (150 minutes) of moderate-intensity aerobic activity every week *and*

Muscle-strengthening activities on two or more days a week that work all major muscle groups (legs, hips, back, abdomen, chest, shoulders, and arms).

Or

Plan B:

One hour and 15 minutes (75 minutes) of vigorous-intensity aerobic activity every week
and
Muscle-strengthening activities on two or more days a week that work all major muscle groups (legs, hips, back, abdomen, chest, shoulders, and arms).

Or

Plan C:

An equivalent mix of moderate and vigorous intensity aerobic activity
and
Muscle-strengthening activities on two or more days a week that work all major muscle groups (legs, hips, back, abdomen, chest, shoulders and arms).

Not all physical activity workouts need to be completed at once. It is acceptable to spread workouts throughout the week as long as the workouts are done at a moderate or vigorous effort for at least 10 minutes per session.

AEROBIC ACTIVITY

Moderate-intensity aerobic activity includes those activities that raise the heart rate and cause a person to break a sweat. (2) (Note: This does not include golf!)

These include:

- Walking fast
- Doing water aerobics
- Riding a bike on level ground or with few hills
- Playing doubles tennis
- Pushing a lawn mower

Vigorous-intensity aerobic activity includes those activities that increase the heart rate so that the patient is breathing hard and fast. At this level, a person will not be able to say more that a few words without pausing for a breath. (2)

- These include:
- Jogging or running

- Swimming laps
- Riding a bike fast or on hills
- Playing singles tennis
- Playing basketball

MUSCLE-STRENGTHENING ACTIVITY

In addition to aerobic activities, muscle-strengthening activities need to be done at least two days a week. These activities should work all the major muscle groups including legs, hips, back, chest, abdomen, shoulders, and arms. The muscle-strengthening activities should be done to the point where it is hard to do another repetition without help; 8–12 repetitions per activity count as one set. Start with one set, working up to two or three sets for more benefits. (2)

These include:

- Lifting weights
- Working with resistance bands
- Doing exercises that use your body weight for resistance (push ups, sit ups)
- Heavy gardening (digging, shoveling)
- Yoga

There are numerous health benefits to staying active. In addition to living longer, healthier lives, research has shown that just 30 minutes a day of activity can contribute to decreased blood pressure, blood glucose control, lower cholesterol, and weight loss.

GET UP AND GO!

- Encourage patients to create their own "action plan" that incorporates different activities that fit with their work and social life.
- At work, stand up and talk on the phone.
- Walk to your co-workers' desks instead of calling or emailing them.
- Walk briskly and take "the long way" when going to meetings.
- Take the stairs.
- Take a walk at lunch (and take your colleagues with you).
- After dinner, get up and take a walk.
- Walk the dog.
- Purchase a pedometer to track your steps during the day. There are even smart phone apps that log your steps. Try to work up to 10,000 steps per day.
- Start a new sport such as bike riding or hiking.
- Stand up and walk around when talking on your cell phone.
- Dance!

Moderate or vigorous physical activity can be done each week. A rule of thumb is that one minute of vigorous activity is equal to two minutes of moderate activity.

BOTTOM LINE

As healthcare providers, it may not be enough to say, "You need to drop 20 pounds." Provide patients with simple, realistic activities to get them moving and help them attain their goals. I saw a sign the other day that read, "Beware—Sitting Is the New Smoking!"

References

1. American College of Sports Medicine. *Reducing sedentary behaviors: sitting less and moving more.* American College of Sports Medicine, 2011. http://www.acsm.org/docs/brochures/reducing-sedentary-behaviors-sitting-less-and-moving-more.pdf.
2. Centers for Disease Control and Prevention. How much physical activity do adults need? Centers for Disease Control and Prevention. http://www.cdc.gov/physicalactivity/everyone/guidelines/adults.html

CHAPTER 35

Diabetes Prevention Plan

D IABETES IS A DEADLY AND COSTLY DISEASE. The risk of death for a person with diabetes is twice the risk of person of similar age who does not have diabetes. (1) Death rates for heart disease and the risk of stroke are approximately 2–4 times higher among adults with diabetes than among those without diabetes. (2)

Average medical expenses are more than twice as high for a person with diabetes as they are for a person without diabetes. (1) In 2007, the estimated cost of diabetes in the United States was $174 billion. That amount included $116 billion in direct medical care costs and $58 billion in indirect costs (from disability, productivity loss, and premature death). (2)

Type 2 diabetes accounts for about 95% of diagnosed diabetes in adults. (1) Rates for type 2 diabetes rise sharply with age for both men and women and for members of all racial and ethnic groups. (1) The prevalence of diagnosed diabetes is about seven times as high among adults ages 65 years or older as among those ages 20–44 years. (1) Race and ethnicity also are risk factors for diabetes. Most minority populations in the United States, including Hispanic Americans and non-Hispanic blacks, have a higher prevalence of diabetes than their white non-Hispanic counterparts. (1)

According to the National Diabetes Surveillance System, the incidence of newly diagnosed diabetes in the United States changed little from 1980 through 1990, but began increasing in 1992. From 1990 through 2010, the annual number of new cases of diagnosed diabetes almost tripled. The rise in the incidence of type 2 diabetes is associated with increases in obesity, a decrease in leisure-time physical activity, and the aging of the U.S. population. (3)

A 2010 CDC study projected that nearly one in three U.S. adults could have diabetes by 2050 if current trends continue. (1) However, several studies have shown that healthy eating and regular physical activity, used with medication if appropriate, can help prevent or delay the onset of type 2 diabetes.

TARGET: PREDIABETES

Having a blood glucose level that is higher than normal but not high enough for a diagnosis of diabetes is called prediabetes. Approximately 33% of U.S. adults have prediabetes and may be at risk of developing type 2 diabetes, heart disease, and stroke. (1) However, it has been found that less than 10% of U.S. adults with prediabetes report that they have been told that they have it. (3)

While having prediabetes is harmful, the progression to type 2 diabetes may be delayed or even prevented. The Diabetes Prevention Program (DPP) conducted a major multicenter clinical research study aimed at discovering whether modest weight loss through dietary changes and increased physical activity or treatment with the oral diabetes drug metformin could prevent or delay the onset of type 2 diabetes in study participants. (4)

The DPP enrolled 3,234 participants from 27 clinical centers around the United States. All participants were overweight and had prediabetes. In addition, 45% of the participants were from minority groups who are typically at high risk of developing diabetes: African American, Alaska Native, American Indian, Asian American, Hispanic/Latino, or Pacific Islander-. (4)

The study participants were randomly divided into three different treatment groups. The first group, the lifestyle intervention group, received intensive training in diet, physical activity, and behavior modification. By eating less fat and fewer calories and exercising for a total of 150 minutes per week, they aimed to lose 7% of their body weight and maintain that loss. (4)

The second group took 850mg of metformin twice daily. The third group received placebo pills instead of metformin. The metformin and placebo groups also received information about diet and exercise but no intensive motivational counseling. (4)

The DPP results showed that participants in the lifestyle intervention group reduced their risk of developing diabetes by 58%. The finding was true across all ethnic groups and for both men and women. Lifestyle changes were particularly effective in participants over 60 years of age, reducing their risk by 71%. Five percent of the lifestyle intervention group developed diabetes each year during the study period in comparison to 11% of those in the placebo group. (4)

Study participants who took metformin reduced their risk of developing diabetes by 31%. Metformin was least effective in people 45 years of age and older. It was most effective in participants 25–44 years old and in those with a body mass index of 35 or higher (60 pounds overweight). About 7.8% of the metformin group developed diabetes each year during the study, compared to 11% of the placebo group.(4)

The results from the DPP indicate that millions of high-risk people can delay or prevent type 2 diabetes by losing weight through regular physical activity and a diet low in fat and calories. Weight loss and physical activity lower the risk of diabetes by improving the body's ability to use insulin and process glucose. The DPP also suggested that metformin could help delay the onset of diabetes. (4)

RISK FACTORS FOR PREDIABETES AND DIABETES (4)

The American Diabetes Association recommends that testing to detect prediabetes and type 2 diabetes be considered in adults without symptoms who are overweight or obese and have one or more additional risk factors for diabetes. In those without risk factors, testing should begin at 45 years of age.

Risk factors include:
✓ Being overweight or obese;
✓ Being 45 years of age or older;
✓ Being physically inactive;
✓ Having a parent, brother, or sister with diabetes;
✓ Having a family background that is African-American, Alaska Native, American Indian, Asian American, Hispanic/Latino, or Pacific Islander;
✓ Giving birth to a baby weighing more than nine pounds or being diagnosed with gestational diabetes;
✓ Having high blood pressure (140/90mmHg or above) or being treated for high blood pressure;
✓ Having an HDL below 35mg/dL or a triglyceride level above 250 mg/dL;
✓ Having polycystic ovary syndrome (PCOS);
✓ Having impaired fasting glucose or impaired glucose tolerance on previous testing;
✓ Having other conditions associated with insulin resistance (severe obesity, acanthosis nigricans); and
✓ Having a history of cardiovascular disease

TAKE ACTION—CREATE A PLAN

• Employ the team approach to treating diabetes. Refer patients and their caregivers to diabetes educators for a complete overview of diabetes and how they can best approach this disease.
• Provide patients with ample resources regarding diabetes. Patient handouts are available on line and many can be reprinted for your use. These resources can

be found on the American Association of Diabetes Educators website at www. diabeteseducator.org

- The Centers for Disease Control and Prevention website also provides many resources and publications:
- www.cdc.gov/diabetes/
- For most patients, telling them to lose weight by eating less will not get them to a goal weight, much less maintain it. Refer patients to a nutritionist who can provide detailed information on dietary changes and restrictions.
- Several online resources are available to assist patients achieve their weight loss goals. Tips for weight loss can be found at www.diabetescare.net and http://diabetes.webmd.com
- Walking 150 minutes each week is a good start to getting in shape, but many patients may need more a more aggressive, specific, and realistic exercise plan. Patients may need the assistance of a personal trainer to get on track.

BOTTOM LINE

The death rate for people with diabetes is twice that for people without diabetes. Weight loss, proper nutrition, and lifestyle changes, including exercise, all help to delay the onset or prevent the disease altogether. Utilize the team approach by including diabetes educators, nutritionists and personal fitness trainers to help patients reach their goals.

References

1. Centers for Disease Control and Prevention. *Diabetes report card 2012.* Atlanta, GA: Centers for Disease Control and Prevention, 2012.
2. Centers for Disease Control and Prevention. *National diabetes factsheet, 2011.* Atlanta, GA: Centers for Disease Control and Prevention, 2012.
3. Geiss LS, James C, Gregg EW, Albright A, et al. Diabetes risk reduction behaviors among U. S. adults with prediabetes. *Am J Prev Med.* 2010 Apr;38(4):403–409. doi: 10.1016/j.amepre.2009.12.029.
4. National Institute of Diabetes and Digestive and Kidney Diseases, National Institutes of Health. National Diabetes Information Clearinghouse. Diabetes Prevention Program. http://diabetes.niddk.nih.gov/dm/pubs/preventionprogram/.

Diabetes Resources

The Wonder Workout provides resources to help people get started with an exercise plan. http://www.prevention.com/

Healthfinder.gov: Provides tools to help people take steps to prevent diabetes.

National Diabetes Information Clearinghouse (NDIC): Provides information to people with diabetes, their families, healthcare professionals, and the public. http://diabetes.niddk.nih.gov

National Diabetes Education Program (NDEP): Provides educational tool kits and multimedia resources for healthcare professionals and diabetes educators. http://ndep.nih.gov/

CHAPTER 36

Prevent What's Preventable

O NE OF MY FAVORITE SAYINGS IS *"Think well of your health. Cure what's curable. Prevent what's preventable. Enjoy the rest."* It is especially true in the area of immunization and vaccination. Immunization has helped to greatly reduce or eliminate many life-threatening infectious diseases in the United States. It is estimated between 2 and 3 million deaths each year are prevented by immunization, (1) making it one of the most cost-effective health investments. According to the Association of State and Territorial Health Officials, every $1 spent on immunizations saves $16 in avoided costs.

Immunizations are accessible to hard-to-reach and vulnerable populations and are delivered effectively through outreach and community services. Vaccination is relatively painless, has few side effects, and does not require any major lifestyle change. (1)

THE AFFORDABLE CARE ACT AND IMMUNIZATIONS

The federal government has long promoted and funded immunizations as a critical public health tool. The Affordable Care Act (ACA) contains new immunization initiatives that focus on additional prevention and public health efforts to increase immunization rates in adults and children. (2) The Affordable Care Act requires new health plans to cover preventive services and eliminate cost-sharing (copayments and deductibles). According to Department of Health and Human Services (HHS) requirements, if an individual or family enrolls in a new health plan on or after September 23, 2010, that plan is required to cover recommended preventive services without charging a deductible, copayment, or coinsurance.

Individuals enrolled in new group or individual health plans will have access to the vaccines recommended by the Advisory Committee on Immunization Practices (ACIP) with no co-payments or other cost-sharing requirements when an in-network provider delivers those services. In 2011, it was estimated that 31 million people in new employer plans and 10 million people in new individual plans benefitted from the new ACA provisions. The number of individuals in employer plans who benefited from the ACA provisions was expected to rise to 78 million by 2013 with a total potential of 88 million Americans whose prevention coverage is expected to improve with the new policy. (3)

Immunizations Covered by the Affordable Care Act: (3)

The immunizations covered by the ACA include:	
For Children and Adolescents • Diphtheria, Tetanus, Pertussis (DTaP) • Haemophilus influenzae Type B • Hepatitis A • Hepatitis B • Human Papillomavirus (HPV) • Inactivated Poliovirus • Influenza • Measles, Mumps, Rubella • Meningococcal • Rotavirus • Tetanus, Diphtheria, Pertussis (Tdap) • Varicella	**For Adults** • Hepatitis A • Hepatitis B • Herpes Zoster • Human Papillomavirus (HPV) • Influenza • Measles, Mumps, Rubella • Meningococcal • Pneumococcal • Tetanus, Diphtheria, Pertussis (Tdap) • Varicella

CHALLENGES AND CONFUSION

The Affordable Care Act immunization plan has created some challenges for patients and providers. The ACA-mandated provision for private insurance and group health plans that ACIP-recommended vaccines are covered at no cost-sharing, translates to over 190 million privately-insured people having access to ACIP-recommended vaccinations and that adult children up to age 26 years who have no health insurance (from 2014, it is regardless of coverage) will have coverage for vaccines. However, no plan is required to cover vaccinations delivered by an out-of-network provider. Plans that do cover out-of-network providers can do so at out-of-network cost-sharing standards. This has also created some problems with patient access to vaccinations since many immunization providers are considered "out-of-network" such as pharmacists and public health departments. (4)

For self-insured group health benefit plans (ERISA plans), the ACA extended many of its standards to include preventive services coverage of all ACIP-recommended vaccines at no cost-sharing. State-regulated private health insurance sold in individual and group health markets prior to March 23, 2010 are "grandfathered" into the ACA. This means that the plan was already in place before the ACA went into effect and is therefore allowed to maintain its old policies for the time being. Routine changes to these grandfathered plans can be made, such as cost adjustments consistent with inflation, addition of new benefits, modest changes to existing benefits, new patient protections, and changes to comply with state and federal requirements. However, grandfathered status will be lost if plans reduce or eliminate existing coverage, increase deductible or co-payments (by more than rate of medical inflation plus 15%), require patients to switch to another grandfathered plan with fewer benefits or higher cost-sharing, or the plan is acquired by or merges with another plan to avoid complying with the ACA. (5)

According to the Kaiser Family Foundation, in 2012 48% of those who received coverage through their jobs were enrolled in a grandfathered health plan and 58% of businesses offering health insurance had at least one grandfathered plan. As of 2014, any remaining grandfathered plans will be considered as providing minimum essential coverage according to the ACA and required to provide preventive services. (6)

There are also certain challenges related to coverage in the states that have opted in to Medicaid expansion. This is due to the fact that expansion and implementation of the exchanges is extremely wide-ranging due to the variability in the states' participation. In states that have opted out of Medicaid expansion, the ACA provisions will not protect traditional Medicaid adult enrollees. This includes 20 million non-elderly persons, including pregnant women, parents/caregivers of dependent children, low-income parents, and working-age adults with disabilities. In this case, immunizations are an optional preventive service for adults.

Despite the changes driven by the ACA, there remains a tremendous lack of vaccination coverage in the United States. According to the Centers for Disease Control and Prevention, in 2011, 62.3% of adults (ages 65+) received pneumococcal vaccine—66.5% were white, 47.6% were black, 43.1% were Hispanic, and 40.3% were Asian. (7) According to the Healthy People 2020 initiatives, the goal for pneumococcal vaccine coverage is 90% for all of these patient populations. (8)

Lack of adult immunization may be related to competing social and economic needs, fewer public health resources, complex vaccine schedules, and limited patient awareness regarding the importance of adult vaccinations. Improving adult immunization rates may depend on improving education and outreach, improving access and ensuring adequate payment for providers. (4)

PAINLESS PREVENTION

- Take advantage of patient education resources available from the CDC and the Immunization Action Coalition.
- Use a team approach to immunization and vaccination by having office staff and other healthcare providers distribute educational materials to patients.
- Use clinical decision support tools (i.e., reminders) to identify patients who need current immunizations.
- Use patient portals to provide current online vaccination records for patients, parents, and caregivers.

- Engage patients by having a discussion regarding actual or perceived adverse reactions and side effects of vaccines, and what to do if they have a reaction or side effect.
- Advocate for an increased number of in-network providers such as pharmacists, school-based clinics, and public health clinics to address access issues.
- Advocate for immunization inclusion for Medicaid patients in states that opt-out of the Medicaid expansion and exchange programs.

BOTTOM LINE

Despite the advancements of the ACA in the payment for immunizations and vaccinations, many gaps remain in coverage, leading to disparity in the actual rate of adult vaccinations. Clinicians are integral in providing patient awareness and access to necessary immunizations and vaccinations.

Resources

Centers for Disease Control and Prevention: http://www.cdc.gov
Immunization Action Coalition: http://www.immunize.org

References

1. World Health Organization. Immunization. *http://www.who.int/topics/immunization/en/*. Accessed May 19, 2013.
2. Wheeler, JB. Immunizations and the affordable care act. LegisBrief of the National Conference of State Legislatures. 2011 April-May; 19(20).
3. U. S. Department of Health and Human Services. The Affordable Care Act and immunization. U. S. Department of Health and Human Services. http://www.hhs.gov/healthcare/facts/factsheets/2010/09/The-Affordable-Care-Act-and-Immunization.html. Accessed June 1, 2013.
4. Tan IJ. The impact of the affordable care act on immunizations—new opportunities and challenges. Immunization Action Coalition. http://www.nhipconference.com/uploads/Impact_of_ACA_on_Immunizations_-_LJ_Tan.pdf
5. U. S. Department of Health and Human Services. Keeping the health plan you have. U. S. Department of Health and Human Services. http://www.healthreform.gov
6. Henry J. Kaiser Foundation. *2012 employer health benefits survey.* Menlo Park, CA: Henry J. Kaiser Foundation, 2012. http://kaiserfamilyfoundation.files.wordpress.com/2013/04/8345.pdf
7. Centers for Disease Control and Prevention. Adult vaccination coverage—United States, 2010. *MMWR Morb Mortal Wkly Rep.* 2012 Feb 3;61(4):66–72.
8. U. S. Department of Health and Human Services. Healthy people 2020. U. S. Department of Health and Human Services. http://www.healthypeople.gov. Accessed October 10, 2013.

CHAPTER 37

Metamorphosis

EARLY CHILDHOOD, MIDDLE CHILDHOOD, AND adolescence represent the three stages of child development. Early childhood (birth to 8 years) is a time of physical, cognitive, and socio-economic development. (1) Middle childhood (ages 6–12 years) is a time when children develop skills for creating lifetime social relationships. Adolescence (ages 10–19) is a stage that includes biological changes of puberty, increasing independence, and normative experimentation. (2) Each of these stages represents a critical period of physical, cognitive, and socio-emotional development leading to a child's healthy development and lifelong learning.

EARLY AND MIDDLE CHILDHOOD

The foundation for a healthy future determined during early and middle childhood. It is during this time that the child learns emotional regulation and attachment, and language and motor skills. (1) During early and middle childhood, many different types of skills emerge, including health literacy, self-discipline, good decision making, healthy eating habits, and conflict resolution. Any stressors that negatively affect the child's development during this time can significantly impact the child's cognitive growth and development. (1)

Early and middle childhood is generally a healthy age; however, children may be at risk for conditions such as asthma, obesity, tooth decay maltreatment, and developmental and behavioral disorders. (1)

ADOLESCENCE

Adolescents (ages 10–19) and young adults (ages 20–24) make up 21% of the U.S. population. (2) Although typically in good health, adolescents may experience serious physical, mental, and social issues and illnesses that may affect their health for years to come, including: homicide, suicide, motor vehicle accidents (drunk driving), substance use/abuse, smoking (tobacco and marijuana), sexually transmitted diseases including HIV, unplanned pregnancies, and homelessness. (2)

Several factors are linked to health outcomes in this age group: (2) 1) proper adult supervision, support, and communication; 2) academic success; 3) distressed neighborhoods and concentrated poverty; and 4) media exposure, (including violence, rape, alcohol, and drug use).

Healthy People 2020 (1,2) has established two important goals and several related objectives to help address the issues faced by children during early childhood, middle childhood, and adolescence.

Goal—Early and Middle Childhood: (1)

Document and track population-based measures of health and well-being for early- and middle-childhood populations in the United States over time.

Objectives: (1)

1. Increase the proportion of children who are ready for school in all five domains of healthy development: physical, social-emotional, approaches to learning, language, and cognitive development.
2. Increase the proportion of parents who use positive parenting and communicate with their doctors or other healthcare professionals about positive parenting.
3. Reduce the proportion of children who have poor quality of sleep.
4. Increase the proportion of elementary, middle, and senior high schools that require school health education.

Goal—Adolescence (2)

Improve the healthy development, health safety, and well-being of adolescents and young adults.

Objectives: (2)

1. Increase the proportion of adolescents who have had a wellness checkup in the past 12 months.
2. Increase the proportion of adolescents who participate in extracurricular and/ or out-of school activities.
3. Increase the proportion of adolescents who are connected to a parent or other positive adult caregiver.
4. Increase the proportion of adolescents and young adults who transition to self-sufficiency from foster care.
5. Increase educational achievement of adolescents and young adults.
6. Increase the proportion of schools with a school breakfast program.
7. Reduce the proportion of adolescents who have been offered, sold, or given an illegal drug on school property.
8. Increase the proportion of adolescents whose parents consider them to be safe at school.

9. Increase the proportion of middle and high schools that prohibit harassment based on a student's sexual orientation or gender identity.
10. Reduce the proportion of public schools with a serious violent incident.
11. Reduce adolescent and young adult perpetration of, and victimization by, crimes.

CHILDHOOD AND ADOLESCENT HEALTH AND WELLBEING

- Provide parents, grandparents, and caregivers with information about positive parenting and creating nurturing and supportive families.
- Provide parents, grandparents, and caregivers with information about community resources for childhood immunization and vaccinations.
- Provide parents, grandparents and caregivers with resource information about their children's learning, development, or behavior.
- Address issues related to poor quality of sleep.
- Be aware of the growing cultural and ethnic diversity and the influence this plays on the health and academic outcomes of adolescents. (2)
- Be aware of the many positive youth development interventions available to today's teens. These have been shown to have a positive impact in creating successful and competent adults. (2)

BOTTOM LINE

Recognizing and understanding the important role that early childhood, middle childhood, and adolescence play in creating healthy adults is vital for healthcare providers. It will enable practitioners to focus on conditions, illnesses, and social issues that can seriously impact a child's ability to play, learn, develop, and grow into a happy, healthy, and successful adult.

References

1. U.S. Department of Health and Human Services. Early and middle childhood. U.S. Department of Health and Human Services. http://www.healthypeople.gov/2020. Accessed June 15, 2013.
2. U. S. Department of Health and Human Services. Adolescent health. U.S. Department of Health and Human Services. *http://www.healthypeople.gov/2020.* Accessed June 15, 2013.

Recommended Resources

American Academy of Pediatrics: www.aap.org/
Big Brothers/Big Sisters of America: www.bbbsa.org
Centers for Disease Control and Prevention—Immunization Schedules: www.cdc.gov
Centers for Disease Control and Prevention—Childhood Development: www.cdc.gov
Centers for Disease Control and Prevention: Parents Portal: www.cdc.gov
Child Development Institute: www.childdevelopmentinfo.com/

Child Trends: www.childtrends.org

Child Welfare League of America—Positive Parenting Tips: www.cwla.org/positiveparenting/

Family Education: www.familyeducation.com

Immunization Action Coalition: www.immunize.org

Kids Online Resources: www.kidsolr.com

National Parent Helpline: www.nationalparenthelpline.org

Netsmartz: www.netsmartz.org

Parenting Help: www.parenting.org

Parenting Resources USA Gov.: www.usa.gov/Topics/Parents.shtml

Positive Parenting: www.positiveparenting.com

SafeKids: www.safekids.com

U.S. Department of Health and Human Services-Child Welfare Information Gateway: www.childwelfare.gov

Zero to Three: www.zerotothree.org

CHAPTER 38

The Complexity of Growing Old

ADULTS OVER THE AGE OF 65 are one of the fastest growing age groups in the United States. This is due, in part, to the first of the "baby boomers" (adults born between 1946 and 1964) turning 65 in 2011. Additionally, it is estimated that over 60% of this group (more than 37 million people) will develop at least one chronic illness by 2030. (1) These chronic conditions include: diabetes mellitus, arthritis, congestive heart failure, and dementia. Chronic conditions are the leading cause of death among older adults. (3)

Dementia, in particular, can drastically impact the cost of care and overall quality of life of older adults. Dementia is the loss of cognitive functioning—thinking remembering, and reasoning—to such an extent that it interferes with a person's daily life. (2) Alzheimer's disease is the most common cause of dementia and is the sixth leading cause of death in adults aged 18 years and older. (4) It is estimated that up to 5.1 million Americans ages 65 years and older have Alzheimer's disease and this number is predicted to double by the year 2050. (5)

As a result of these chronic conditions, many older adults experience a high rate emergency room visits, hospitalizations, and nursing home or rehabilitation stays.

HEALTHY PEOPLE 2020

Preventive healthcare services for older adults are addressed in two of the new goals for Healthy People 2020. (2)

These goals are:

1. Improve the health, function, and quality of life of older adults.
   * Increase the proportion of older adults who use the Welcome to Medicare benefit.
   * Increase the proportion of older adults who are up to date on a core set of clinical preventive services.
   * Increase the proportion of older adults with one or more chronic health conditions who report confidence in managing their conditions.

- Increase the proportion of older adults who receive Diabetes Self-Management Benefits.
- Reduce the proportion of older adults who have moderate to severe functional limitations.
- Increase the proportion of older adults with reduced physical or cognitive function who engage in light, moderate, or vigorous leisure-time physical activities.
- Increase the proportion of the healthcare workforce with geriatric certification.

2. Reduce the morbidity and costs associated with, and maintain or enhance the quality of life for persons with dementia, including Alzheimer's disease.
   - Increase the proportion of persons with diagnosed Alzheimer's disease and other dementias or their caregiver, who are aware of the diagnosis.
   - Reduce the proportion of preventable hospitalizations in persons with diagnosed Alzheimer's disease and other dementias.

In addition to the Healthy People 2020 goals, the Patient Protection and Affordable Care Act of 2010 includes provisions related to relevant Medicare services for older adults. These older adults may need many different healthcare services and require professional expertise that meets their needs. Federal government agencies and programs that target chronic illness, especially in minorities and the underserved, can help to improve physician, hospital, and nursing home care. However, according to the Centers for Medicare and Medicaid Services (CMS) preventive services for these chronic illnesses are *underused*, especially among certain racial and ethnic groups.

PREVENTIVE CARE IN OLDER ADULTS

- Use of preventive health services can greatly improve health outcomes in older adults. Provide patients with necessary information so they can access community agencies, internet resources, local programs, and other social services to help them better manage their chronic conditions and long-term needs effectively.
- The ability to self-manage chronic diseases can improve health outcomes. Refer patients to diabetes educators, lipid management clinics, anticoagulation clinics, pharmacist medication management clinics, pain management specialists, and congestive heart failure, and other chronic disease management resources.
- Participation in physical activity (including strength training) has been shown to improve health outcomes in older adults. Refer patients to community organizations that provide guided and age-appropriate physical fitness training programs.
- Refer patients with dementia to specialists for assistance with initiation of proper medication therapy if necessary.

- Provide caregivers of patients with dementia, resources for respite care and financial assistance (if necessary).
- Assess whether housing or transportation is impacting the ability of your older patients to access the care they need. Refer to community resources for housing and transportation if necessary.
- Providers (or office staff) may need to intervene in the care of the older adult by assisting with coordination of care, helping older adult manage their own care, and provide training for the people who care for older adults.

BOTTOM LINE

Despite numerous preventive care initiatives for older adults, there is an under use of government programs aimed at treating chronic illness. It is up to the provider to be aware of these programs and inform the patients and their caregivers of these initiatives. Office staff may be instrumental in assisting with referrals and coordination of services to ensure much needed care.

References

1. American Hospital Association. *When I'm 64: how boomers will change healthcare.* Washington, DC: American Hospital Association; 2007.
2. U. S. Department of Health and Human Services. Healthy people 2020. U. S. Department of Health and Human Services. www.healthypeople.gov. Accessed June 16, 2013.
3. Kramarow E, Lubitz J, Lentzner H, Gorina Y. Trends in the health of older Americans. *Health Aff (Millwood).* 2007 Sep-Oct;26(5):1417–1425.
4. Xu J, Kochanek KD, Murphy SL, Tejada-Vera B. Deaths: Preliminary data for 2007. *National Vital Statistics Reports.* Hyattsville, MD: National Center for Health Statistics, 2009.
5. Hebert LE, Scherr PA, Bienias JL, et al. Alzheimer disease in the US population: prevalence estimates using the 2000 census. *Arch Neurol.* 2003 Aug;60(8):1119–1122.

Resources

Healthy Aging Topics

Centers for Disease Control and Prevention—Health information for older adults
www.cdc.gov/aging/

NIH Senior Health—Health and wellness information for older adults from the National Institutes of Health
www.nihseniorhealth.gov/

National Institute on Aging—Research-based information and resources related to health and aging
www.nia.nih.gov

Administration on Aging—Health, prevention, and wellness program
www.aoa.gov

CHAPTER 39

Health Literacy

EFFECTIVE COMMUNICATION IS DEFINED AS the "successful joint establishment of meaning wherein patients and healthcare providers exchange information, enabling patients to participate actively in their care from admission through discharge and ensuring that the responsibilities of both patients and providers arc understood." (8) Easier said than done! Providing complex health information to patients and ensuring that they understand it is critical to successful healthcare management; however, this requires thorough and comprehensive communication between providers, patients, and their caregivers.

The Centers for Medicare and Medicaid Services (CMS) has included the "Use of certified Electronic Health Record technology (CEHRT) to identify patient-specific education resources and provide those resources to the patient if appropriate" as a core objective for eligible professionals.

Stage 1: More than 10% of all unique patients seen by the EP are provided patient-specific education resources.

Stage 2: Patient-specific education resources identified by CEHRT are provided to patient for more than 10% of all unique patients with office visits seen by the EP during the EHR reporting period.

Effective communication helps bridge the verbal, social and cultural gap between the doctor and patient and goes a long way to promote the doctor-patient partnership both with the patient themselves and their families. (1) However, successful communication can only be accomplished when providers understand and integrate the information gleaned from patients and when patients comprehend accurate, timely, complete, and unambiguous messages from providers in a way that enables them to participate responsibly in their care. (8)

HEALTH LIT 101

Optimal healthcare outcomes depend on the provider's capability to communicate complicated information with his or her patients. However, limited patient health literacy has been and continues to be an obstacle in providing effective patient care.

The term "health literacy" has been coined to describe the individual patient's ability to comprehend and act on complex medical information. It is "the capacity to obtain, interpret and understand basic health information and services needed to make appropriate health care decisions." (2)

It is estimated that nearly 90 million U.S. adults have inadequate health literacy skills, (3) and this is likely to increase as the population ages (4) and the treatment of chronic illness becomes more complex.

The 2003 National Assessment of Adult Literacy defined health literacy as (5):

- **Below basic**—Patient can circle the date of a medical appointment on an appointment slip, but is unable to understand a simple pamphlet about pre-test instructions.
- **Basic**—Patient can locate one piece of information in a short document or can understand a simple patient education handout.
- **Intermediate**—Patient is able to determine healthy weight for a person on a body mass index chart and can interpret prescription and over-the-counter drug labels.
- **Proficient**—Patient is able to define medical terms from complex document, can calculate share of employee's health insurance costs, and has the skills needed to manage health and prevent disease.

The impact of low health literacy on readmission rates and the overall quality of healthcare is significant. Low health literacy has been found to be an independent risk factor for worse outcomes, including increased mortality, lower satisfaction with care, lower quality of care, poorer patient safety, and higher healthcare costs. (6)

In a multi-site study of primary care patients, it was found that approximately half (46.3%) were unable to read and correctly state one or more of the label instruction on five common prescriptions. Misunderstanding was higher in patients with marginal and low literacy, yet 37.7% of patients with adequate literacy skills misunderstood at least one of the label instructions. (7) For example, among the patients correctly stating the instruction "Take two tablets by mouth twice daily" (84.3%), one-third were unable to state the correct number of pills to take each day. This study concluded that even though patients were able to read the label instructions correctly, they could not accurately state the number of pills to be taken suggesting that numeracy may be a more difficult literacy task than reading the words. (7)

THE FOUR QUESTIONS YOUR PATIENTS NEED TO ASK
(Every time they get a new medication)

Having patients ask four simple questions can help them get the information they need quickly and take their new medications safely. These four questions are:

1. **What is the Name of the drug?** Patients should know both the generic and the brand name of the drug. If you are prescribing a generic, the pharmacist should type both the brand name and generic name on the prescription label to prevent confusion and avoid duplication. For example: lisinopril, generic for Zestril.
2. **What is it Used for?** Clinicians can write the use, or reason for taking the drug, on the prescription itself (or electronic prescription) and the pharmacist will then print it on the prescription label. For example, "Take one tablet every day for high blood pressure." This helps patients and caregivers remember what a medication is for.
3. **How should I Take it?** Patients should know exactly how to take the medication before they leave the hospital, doctor's office, or pharmacy. This includes appropriate time of day, with or without food, and with or without other medications.
4. **What are the Side effects?** Patients should be told common side effects of a new drug and what they should do if they have a side effect. Knowing what to expect from a new drug and what to do can prevent unnecessary office or emergency room visits.

To make it easy, patients should be told to remember the acronym: **N.U.T.S.**—Name, Use, Take, and Side effects. They should not leave the hospital, physician's office, or pharmacy without asking and understanding the answers to these four questions.

Have patients or their caregivers write down the information they are given so they will not forget it after they get home. Have patients repeat the information back to you (teach back), so you can ensure they understand what had been said. Also, have patients ask the pharmacist for written information about the drug and urge them to ask questions about any information they may not remember or fully understand.

"I DIDN'T WANT HIM TO THINK I WAS STUPID."

James was an elderly gentleman who had been admitted to the Cardiac Care Unit (CCU) for a life-threatening cardiac arrhythmia. His cardiologist and CCU nurses worked around the clock for nearly a week to restore James back to health. This included stabilizing him on a new medication regimen.

Following his stay in the CCU and several more days on the cardiac floor, James was ready to be discharged. He was being given several new prescriptions, including amiodarone and warfarin. The prescriptions were sent electronically to James' pharmacy for him to pick up on his way home.

Prior to leaving the hospital, James's doctor went to see him. He sat at the bedside and slowly went over every new drug that he was prescribing for James, specifically the amiodarone and warfarin. He told James what the new drugs were for and how James should take them at home. He told James about the side effects and what he should do if they occurred. He also told James that the pharmacist would be coming to see him before he went home to briefly go over his new blood thinner and to set up an appointment in three days to monitor the effects of his new medications. The pharmacist would be working closely with the doctor to make sure that James was taking the new drugs correctly and that he was responding to the therapy as planned. James acknowledged what his doctor had been saying by nodding his head and smiling.

Three days later, James came to the anticoagulation clinic to be seen by the pharmacist for follow up on his warfarin therapy. The pharmacist reviewed the INR that had been drawn that day and was confused. The INR indicated that no blood thinner had been taken in the past several days. The pharmacist compared the days' reading to the last one from the hospital and there was definitely a problem. In discussing the new medicines with James, it became apparent that James had not been taking the warfarin, amiodarone, or any of the new medications at all. The pharmacist called the doctor, who immediately came to the anticoagulation clinic to see James.

When James' doctor asked him how he was taking the new medications, James said that he did not know he had any new medications. He did not know that he was supposed to go to the pharmacy after leaving the hospital. In fact, he had just gone home and started taking his old medications as before.

In a very kind way, James' doctor asked James why he did not speak up and tell him that he did not understand the directions he was giving him. James said that he was just too embarrassed to admit that he did not understand anything that the doctor had told him. He said, "I just didn't want you to think I was stupid."

James was readmitted to the hospital to resume amiodarone and warfarin therapy. He was admitted for three days until he was again stabilized on these medications. His provider again gave James discharge instructions. However, this time James was also counseled by the pharmacist who went over all of James' medications and provided a list of drugs that he should be taking at home. James was also referred to the anticoagulation clinic for monitoring of his warfarin and given the exact date and time of his next appointment. James left the hospital with written directions and the phone number of the doctor and the pharmacist to call if he had any questions.

CLEAR UP CONFUSION BEFORE THEY LEAVE

- Limit the use of medical terms and jargon. Even if the patients act like they understand, they may misinterpret what you say.
- Use multiple forms of communication, including verbal, written, and visual, to enhance the patients' knowledge of the information being given to them.

- Ask the patient, "What questions do you have for me?" rather than "Do you have any questions?"
- Confirm patient understanding by using the "teach-back" method. Ask them to restate to you in their own words what they have been told to do (i.e., "Tell me exactly how you are going to take this medication and what it is for.")
- Use educational materials that meet health literacy needs. Materials should be written at fifth-grade or lower reading level. Review and revise current materials if necessary.
- Revise patient education materials to meet the needs of all patients. Divide complex information into bullet points, enlarge the font to assist with vision difficulties, simplify the layout, and revise written information to improve readability. (8)
- Provide an interpreter if necessary, even if the hospital has materials written in the patient's native language.
- Engage caregivers and notify them about ongoing communication issues. Encourage families to ask questions and to write down questions for all staff involved in the discharge or transition of care.

BOTTOM LINE

Low health literacy is a common yet very serious problem. It is associated with poorer health outcomes, lower satisfaction, and adverse patient safety events. Providers should use appropriate written and other means of communication to ensure safe healthcare, reduce readmissions, and enhance the patient-provider relationship. Finally, have patients learn the four questions they need to ask by remembering the acronym NUTS: Name, Use, Take, and Side effects.

References

1. Sarkar U, Schillinger D. Literacy and patient care. http://www.uptodate.com/contents/literacy-and-patient-care. Accessed February 10, 2013.
2. U. S. Department of Health and Human Services. Healthy People 2010: health communication. U. S. Department of Health and Human Services. http://www.healthypeople.gov. Accessed February 10, 2013.
3. Nielsen-Bohlman L, Panzer A, Kindig D, et al. *Health Literacy: A Prescription to End Confusion.* Washington, D.C.: National Academies Press, 2004.
4. Gazmararian JA, Baker DW, Williams MV, et al. Health literacy among Medicare enrollees in a managed care organization. *JAMA.* 1999 Feb 10; 281(6):545–551.
5. Institute of Education Sciences. *2003 National Assessment of Adult Literacy.* Washington, D.C.: U. S. Department of Education, 2003.
6. Baker DW, Parker RM, Williams MV, Clark WS. Health literacy and the risk of hospital admission. *J Gen Intern Med.* 1998 Dec;13(12):791–798.

7. Davis TC, Wolf MS, Bass PF 3rd, Thompson JA, et al. Literacy and misunderstanding prescription drug labels. *Ann Intern Med.* 2006 Dec 19; 145(12):887–894. Epub 2006 Nov 29. Literacy and misunderstanding prescription drug labels.

8. The Joint Commission. *Advancing Effective Communication, Cultural Competence, and Patient-and Family-Centered Care: A Roadmap for Hospitals.* Oakbrook Terrace, IL: The Joint Commission, 2010.

PATIENT INFORMATION MATERIALS

The following websites and resources are provided for educational purposes only and are not to be used in place of medical advice, diagnosis, treatment recommendations, or referrals to practitioners.

For Drug Information

MedlinePlus: A service of the U.S. National Library of Medicine and the National Institutes of Health that provides information on prescription and over-the-counter medications—www.nlm.nih.gov/medlineplus/druginformation.html

U.S. Food and Drug Administration Center for Drug Evaluation and Research: Provides information on prescription and over-the-counter medications, consumer drug information, reports, and publications—www.fda.gov/cder. Main FDA for general inquiries: 888-INFO-FDA (888-463-6332). Drug Information: 301-827-4570. To submit a report about Adverse Drug Reaction: Medwatch: 800-FDA-1088.

Drugs.com: Provides information on nearly 24,000 different prescription drugs, over-the-counter meds, and natural products, including pill identification, drug interaction checker, and side effects—www.drugs.com.

United States Pharmacopeia (USP): An official public standards-setting authority for all prescription and over-the-counter medicines and other health-care products—www.usp.org.

NCCAM Clearinghouse: Provides information on complementary and alternative medicine—www.nccam.nih.gov. Toll-free in the United States: 888-644-6226. TTY (for deaf and hard-of-hearing callers): 1866-464-3615. E-mail: info@nccam.nih.gov.

PubMed: A service of the National Library of Medicine (NLM), it provides summaries of articles from scientific and medical journals—www.ncbi.nlm.nih.gov/entrez.

Cochrane Collaboration Database: Summarizes the results of clinical trials on healthcare treatments. (Summaries are free. Full-text articles require a subscription.)— www.cochrane.org.

Verified Internet Pharmacy Practice Sites (VIPPS): The VIPPS symbol signifies public accountability of the pharmacy and the commitment to the patient's health and safety. Check out this website before ordering medications online—www. nabp.net/programs/accreditation/vipps/.

Quality Check: The Joint Commission on the Accreditation of Healthcare Organization's search engine to locate accredited healthcare organizations in the United States. Visitors can search by city and state, by name, or by zip code—www. qualitycheck.org/consumer/searchQCR.aspx.

Hospital Compare: Allows patients to compare and find the best hospitals in the United States based on several indicators—www.hospitalcompare.hhs.gov.

Healthgrades: A private organization designed to provide ratings and profiles of hospitals, nursing homes, and physicians—www.healthgrades.com.

Consumers Advancing Patient Safety (CAPS): Promotes a partnership between patients and doctors—www.patientsafety.org/.

Medication Safety Websites

These websites focus on educating the consumer and the healthcare provider about medication errors and patient safety.

- ✓ Institute for Safe Medication Practices—www.ismp.org
- ✓ The Joint Commission on the Accreditation of Healthcare Organizations—www.jointcommission.org
- ✓ Agency for Healthcare Research and Quality—Medical Error and Patient Safety—www.ahrq.gov
- ✓ American Society of Health-System Pharmacists—Patient Safety Resource Center—www.ashp.org/patientsafety
- ✓ Citizens for Patient Safety—http://citizensforpatientsafety.org/
- ✓ Institute for Healthcare Improvement—www.ihi.org
- ✓ Institute of Medicine—www.iom.edu
- ✓ National Patient Safety Foundation—www.npsf.org
- ✓ National Coordinating Council on Medication Error Reporting and Prevention—www.nccmerp.org
- ✓ National Council on Patient Information and Education—talkaboutrx.org/
- ✓ National Quality Forum—www.qualityforum.org/Home.aspx
- ✓ Patient Safety and Quality Healthcare—www.psqh.com
- ✓ Partnership for Patient Safety—http://p4ps.net/Home.html/
- ✓ Safety Leaders—www.safetyleaders.org

CHAPTER 40

Social Determinants of Health

- Why do some people get the healthcare they need and others don't?
- What determines why some people are healthy and others are not?
- What role do personal, social, economic, and environmental factors play in obtaining optimum healthcare?

To answer these questions, one needs to identify and acknowledge the impact of social factors on an individual's health. Social determinants of health are factors in the environment in which people are born, live, learn, work, play, worship, and age that affect a wide range of health, functioning, and quality-of-life outcomes and risks. (1) Additionally, social engagement, a sense of security and well-being, as well as availability and access to medical resources can significantly impact health outcomes. (1) One study suggests that there may be up to a 20-year gap in life expectancy between the most- and least-advantaged populations in the United States. (2)

In response to this disparity, Healthy People 2020 has adopted the goal of " Creating social and physical environments that promote good health for all." (1) The aim is to reduce the inequality in access to healthcare, social and economic opportunities, and community resources between different factions of American society. It also aims to provide quality schools, safe workplaces, clean air and water, and healthy food, and to optimize social interactions and relationships. These social factors may impact why some Americans are healthier than others and why Americans are not as healthy as they should be.

Healthy People 2020 has created five key areas in addressing the social determinants of health. (1) These are:

1. **Economic Stability:** Decrease poverty, unemployment, and homelessness.
2. **Education:** Increase high school graduation rates and enrollment in higher education, provide safe school environments, and institute school policies that incorporate the promotion of healthy behaviors.
3. **Social and Community Context:** Improve the family structure and social cohesion; reduce discrimination, incarceration, and institutionalization.
4. **Health and Health Care:** Improve access to health services, including preventive care and primary care, and improve health technology.

5. **Neighborhood and Built Environment:** Improve the quality of housing and environmental conditions, reduce crime and violence, and improve access to healthy foods.

In addition to the efforts of Healthy People 2020, the World Health Organization (WHO) has created the Commission on Social Determinants of Health. The goal of this commission is to eliminate health inequities throughout the world.

It strives to do this by:

- Improving the conditions of daily life—the circumstances in which people are born, grow, live, work, and age.
- Tackling the inequitable distribution of power, money, and resources—the structural drivers of the conditions of daily life—globally, nationally and locally.
- Measuring the problem, evaluating the action, expanding the knowledge base, developing a workforce that is trained in the social determinants of health, and raising public awareness about the social determinants of health impacting overall healthcare. (3)

The Centers for Disease Control and Prevention (CDC) has also created several initiatives, committees, and work groups tasked with addressing this issue. The mission of these groups is to help eliminate health disparities for vulnerable populations, including those defined by race/ethnicity, socioeconomic status, geography, gender, age, disability status, and other at-risk populations. (4)

With global, national, and local efforts solidly underway, why is it that inequities in healthcare exist in this country and what can be done to correct this? Additionally, what role should medical providers play when societal factors extend beyond traditional healthcare boundaries?

REMEDY FOR HEALTH INEQUALITIES

- Addressing social determinants of health involves not only providing medical care and public health systems, but extends outside of usual healthcare boundaries.
- Collaboration of multiple areas, including education, housing, labor, justice, transportation, agriculture, and environment, will be necessary to successfully negotiate the issues surrounding social determinants of health. (5)
- Monitoring for potential social determinants that could lead to poor health outcomes should occur during the initial encounter with the provider.
- Monitoring for potential inequities in access to care should occur in all patient encounters.

- Disparities in outcomes may be due to social factors and should be tracked for possible system or policy changes.
- A "health in all policies" strategy should be applied to close gaps in policy and decision making in all areas of healthcare. (6)

BOTTOM LINE

Social determinants of health, such as poverty, lack of access to healthcare, poor education, and racism, are underlying factors of health inequities leading to poor health outcomes. Changes must be made to these underlying societal issues before a significant and sustained change can be made to the American healthcare system.

References

1. U. S. Department of Health and Human Services. Social determinants of health. U. S. Department of Health and Human Services. http://healthypeople.gov/2020. Accessed June 2, 2013.
2. Murray CJL, Michaud C, Mckenna MT, Marks JS. *U.S. Patterns of Mortality by County and Race: 1965–1994*. Atlanta and Boston: U.S. Centers for Disease Control and Prevention and Harvard School of Public Health; 1998.
3. World Health Organization Commission on Social Determinants of Health. *Closing the Gap in a Generation: Health Equity Through Action on the Social Determinants of Health. Final report of the Commission on Social Determinants of Health*. Geneva, Switzerland: World Health Organization, 2008.
4. Centers for Disease Control and Prevention. *Social determinants of health. Centers for Disease Control and Prevention*. http://www.origin.glb.cdc.gov/social determinants/FAQ.html. Accessed June 1, 2013.
5. Jones, CP. *Social Determinants of Equity and Social Determinants of Health*. Atlanta, GA: Centers for Disease Control and Prevention.
6. European Observatory on Health Systems and Policies. *Health in All Policies: Prospects and Potentials*. Helsinki, Finland: Finnish Ministry of Social Affairs and Health. http://www.euro.who.int/__data/assets/pdf_file/0003/109146/E89260.pdf. Accessed June 1, 2013.

INDEX